A Practical Guide to Early Intervention and Family Support

of related interest

Adult Drug Problems, Children's Needs
Assessing the Impact of Parental Drug Use
Second Edition
Joy Barlow, Di Hart and Jane Powell
ISBN 978 1 90939 125 3
eISBN 978 1 90939 129 1

Putting Analysis Into Child and Family Assessment
Undertaking Assessments of Need
Third Edition
Ruth Dalzell and Emma Sawyer
ISBN 978 1 90939 123 9
eISBN 978 1 90939 127 7

Social Work with Troubled Families
A Critical Introduction
Edited by Keith Davies
ISBN 978 1 84905 549 9
eISBN 978 0 85700 974 6

Practical Guide to Child Protection
The Challenges, Pitfalls and Practical Solutions
Joanna Nicolas
ISBN 978 1 84905 586 4
eISBN 978 1 78450 032 0

Direct Work with Family Groups
Simple, Fun Ideas to Aid Engagement, Assessment and Enable Positive Change
Audrey Tait and Helen Wosu
ISBN 978 1 84905 554 3
eISBN 978 0 85700 986 9

Risk in Child Protection Work
Frameworks for Practice
Martin C. Calder
ISBN 978 1 84905 479 9
eISBN 978 0 85700 858 9

A Practical Guide to Early Intervention and Family Support

Assessing Needs and Building Resilience in Families Affected by Parental Mental Health Problems or Substance Misuse

Emma Sawyer and Sheryl Burton

Foreword by Alison O'Sullivan

Jessica Kingsley *Publishers*
London and Philadelphia

Adaptation of text from pp.40–6: 'The Cycle of Change' from *Changing for Good* by James O. Prochaska, John C. Norcross and Carlo C. Diclemente. Copyright © 1994 by James O. Prochaska, John C. Norcross and Carlo C. Diclemente. Reprinted by permission of HarperCollins Publishers.

Miller, W. R. and Rollnick, S. (2002) *Motivational Interviewing: Preparing People for Change*. New York: Guilford Press. Used with permission of Guilford Press.

The Family Star™ on page 122 is reproduced with permisssion.
Family Star™ (2nd Edition) © Triangle Consulting Social Enterprise Ltd.

First edition published in 2009 by National Children's Bureau
Second edition published in 2012 by National Children's Bureau
Previously published as Building Resilience in Families Under Stress

This edition first published in 2016 by National Children's Bureau
an imprint of Jessica Kingsley Publishers
73 Collier Street
London N1 9BE, UK
and
400 Market Street, Suite 400
Philadelphia, PA 19106, USA

www.jkp.com

Copyright © National Children's Bureau 2009, 2012, 2016

Foreword copyright © Alison O'Sullivan 2016

Front cover image source: iStockphoto®. The cover image is for illustrative purposes only, and any person featuring is a model.

Library of Congress Cataloging in Publication Data
Sawyer, Emma (Sociologist)
 [Building resilience in families under stress]
 A practical guide to early intervention and family support : assessing needs and building resilience in families affected by parental mental health and substance misuse / Emma Sawyer and Sheryl Burton.
    pages cm
 Revised edition of the authors' Building resilience in families under stress, 2012.
 Includes bibliographical references and index.
 ISBN 978-1-909391-21-5
 1. Dysfunctional families--Services for--Great Britain. 2. Family social work--Great Britain. I. Burton, Sheryl. II. Sawyer, Emma (Sociologist) Building resilience in families under stress. III. Title.
 HV700.G7S29 2015
  362.2--dc23
                              2015027309

British Library Cataloguing in Publication Data
A CIP catalogue record for this book is available from the British Library

ISBN 978 1 90939 121 5
eISBN 978 1 90939 130 7

Printed and bound in Great Britain

NCB's vision is of a society in which children and young people contribute, are valued, and their rights respected. Our mission is to improve children and young people's experiences and life chances, reducing the impact of inequalities. NCB aims to:

- reduce inequalities of opportunity in childhood
- ensure children and young people can use their voice to improve their lives and the lives of those around them
- improve perceptions of children and young people
- enhance the health, learning, experiences and opportunities of children and young people
- encourage the building of positive and supportive relationships for children and young people with families, carers, friends and communities
- provide leadership through the use of evidence and research to improve policy and practice.

NCB has adopted and works within the UN Convention on the Rights of the Child.

Contents

List of practice examples

Foreword

by Alison O'Sullivan

Families in need of additional help and support remain high on the national policy agenda with the expansion of the government's Troubled Families programme alongside other initiatives such as the recently established, cross-departmental taskforce to 'transform child protection'.[1] While these developments, and others in local services, are not specifically focused on families affected by parental substance misuse or mental health problems, too many local authorities across the country are reporting rising numbers of families experiencing complex difficulties linked to these issues.

The impact on children of all ages can be both serious and long lasting so there is an urgent and essential need for all public services to respond as quickly and effectively as possible to the needs of families affected by these issues. All parents will want to look after their children, however their ability to provide the necessary levels of care and support can be significantly impeded by poor mental well-being and physical addictions.

The stigma surrounding mental illnesses and substance misuse can prevent parents from seeking the help that they need, and this, combined with delays in assessments of need, can compound the situation. It is therefore vitally important that the professionals working with those affected by these issues are equipped with the right knowledge, skills and attitudes to work constructively with families and prioritise children's needs.

The concept of resilience and how to foster it has proved useful for practitioners working in this area, offering, as it does, a dynamic and proactive approach. When combined with careful analysis and the sound professional judgement of the interaction between risk and protective factors, it can help forge better responses in practice with individual families but also in service development and provision.

---

1   See www.gov.uk/government/news/pm-announces-new-taskforce-to-transform-child-protection

This handbook has been designed to meet the needs of practitioners across a wide range of agencies, including of course local authorities, and it should help those working in these complex circumstances to translate the concept of resilience into practice reality. It provides models, frameworks and crucially real examples in order to assist professionals in their task of helping families with complex needs to better meet their children's needs.

Alison O'Sullivan, President of the Association of Directors of Children's Services and Director of Children's Services in Kirklees

Acknowledgements

We would like to thank the now closed Parenting Fund for funding the Building Resilience project and the publication of the first edition of this handbook.

The first edition was written by Emma Sawyer, Senior Development Officer at the National Children's Bureau (NCB), with assistance from Sheryl Burton, Director, and Steve Howell, Information Development Officer, Social Inclusion department, NCB. The second edition was updated by Sheryl Burton, with specific contributions from Emma Sawyer, Zoe Renton, Head of Policy, NCB and Rhian Beynon, Head of Policy and Campaigns, Family Action, with assistance from Kate Thomas, Projects Assistant. This third edition has been updated by Sheryl Burton and Emma Sawyer with specific contributions from Zoe Renton and Keith Clements, Policy Officer, NCB, with assistance from Kate Thomas.

Thanks to all the original contributors of practice examples and to the agencies and professionals who participated in the Building Resilience project by attending workshops and sharing ideas, experiences and practice examples, including the following workshop speakers: David Bailey, Amynta Cardwell, Donald Forrester, Tracey Hicks, Ellen Marks. Rose De Paeztron, Christine Puckering, Wendy Robinson, Catherine Shaw, Jo Tunnard, and Michele Wates.

Thanks to advisory group members for their time and expertise in the planning, development and undertaking of the project and contributing their ideas for the first edition of this handbook. Job titles and even names of advisory group members may have changed in the intervening years but at the time of the project and the publication of the first edition they were:

Jo Tunnard (Chair; and Writer, Researcher and Consultant) Debbie Cowley (Director of Practice Development, Parenting UK) Ruth Dalzell (Freelance Trainer and Consultant)

Rose De Paeztron (Head of Strategic Development, Family Welfare Association)

Dr Donald Forrester (Reader in Child Welfare and Director of the Child and Family Welfare Research Unit, Bedfordshire University)

Eva Geser (Coordinator, Families and Prevention Programme, Adfam)

Brendan McLoughlin and Emma Raver (London Development Centre for Mental Health) Suzanne Murray (Parenting Policy Officer, Alcohol Concern)

Michele Wates (Writer, Researcher, Campaigner).

The views expressed in the handbook are those of the authors and not necessarily those of all steering group members.

Introduction

This is the third edition of this handbook, which, like the editions before it, seeks to illuminate and provide practical assistance to frontline practitioners and managers grappling with some of the most complex and persistent difficulties and dilemmas facing professionals across a range of adult and children's services – how to work effectively and achieve better and lasting outcomes and life experiences for children and families affected by parental substance misuse or parental mental health problems or both. The original handbook emerged from the National Children's Bureau (NCB) project, Building Resilience and Supporting Relationships in Families under Stress, which ran from 2004 to 2006. The project's aim was to explore how relevant practitioners and professionals could support parenting more effectively in families affected by parental substance misuse and/or mental health problems. It provided what was then a rare opportunity for a diverse group of practitioners and professionals to come together – from adult, children and family services in the voluntary and statutory sectors – to consider and work on key issues. This process was interesting and informative for those involved and led to many participants developing and undertaking action plans locally to improve services. The handbook sought to bring the issues and points raised to readers concerned with improving the support provided by agencies to families with multiple and complex difficulties. While the policy and service context has changed considerably since then, with a greater emphasis at strategic and practice levels on working across the interfaces of adults' and children's services, challenges persist along with the need for building the resilience of children, families and those who support them.

Who is this handbook for?

The handbook is for practitioners and managers who are directly or indirectly involved in the provision of statutory or voluntary services to any family members affected by parental mental health problems, parental substance misuse or alcohol misuse, or a combination of these, who are working in:

- statutory and voluntary adult services, such as mental health or drug and alcohol teams
- statutory and voluntary children's services
- family-based services, including Troubled Families teams or other Early Help services, children's or family centres, child and adolescent mental health services (CAMHS), family group conferencing teams and parental mental health services
- universal services, such as health or education settings
- specialist services, such as drug treatment centres, psychiatric services or services aimed specifically at black and ethnic minority children and families or those provided to young carers
- any of the above services as commissioners or planners
- places other than the above but who have a professional, personal or academic interest in 'what helps' in supporting children and families in these circumstances.
- social work students and social work educators.

How can it be used?

The handbook can be used by practitioners across a range of agencies to assist with reflection and consideration of the impacts on children and families affected by parental substance misuse and mental health problems, how the negative impact of such circumstances can be minimised, protective elements boosted and what interventions, support, knowledge or resources may be helpful. It is designed to be used flexibly to meet a variety of needs and thus can be read cover to cover or dipped into whenever a section or practice example becomes particularly relevant. The practice examples are listed on page 9.

What is in the handbook?

Chapter 1 provides some contextual information relating to parental substance misuseand mental health problems in families, including: definitions; prevalence; and the policy and legislative context. It ends with a brief discussion of current service responses in the UK for families in these circumstances.

Chapter 2 draws on literature and research to explore the potential impact on children and families of parental mental health problems and/or substance misuse, using the domains of the *Framework for the Assessment of Children in Need and their Families* (Department of Health 2000).

Chapter 3 explores the concept of resilience and highlights factors that can bolster families' abilities to meet their children's needs and improve the life chances for young people in adverse circumstances.

Chapter 4 explores some of the barriers to the provision of effective support to families affected by parental substance misuse or parental mental health problems.

Part One examines difficulties and barriers at the practice level and Part Two examines them at the strategic and service planning level.

Chapter 5 considers 'what's needed' in order to make service responses more appropriate and supportive to families in these circumstances at the individual practice level.

Chapter 6 considers 'what's needed' in order to make service responses more appropriate and supportive to families in these circumstances at the strategic level of service planning and organisation.

Chapter 7 provides a concluding summary of the key messages arising out of chapters 1–6.

The Further Resources section provides information about relevant organisations and resources that may assist in developing planning and practice.

The practice examples

The practice examples come from a range of sources; many describe approaches taken by agencies that participated in the original Building Resilience project, while others have come to our attention more recently. We have not been in a position to assess directly or to validate the effectiveness of these approaches, but they do seem to us to demonstrate potentially useful ideas and approaches.

1

Context, legislation and policy

A large number of families are affected by parental substance misuse, parental mental health problems or both. Apart from the direct effects upon the adults and children within those families, the indirect impact on the various relevant services working with them is 'pervasive, hidden and under recognised' (Kearney, Levin and Rosen 2003a, p.7). This chapter argues that many parents with these problems remain concerned for the welfare of their children and can cope with their parental responsibilities given adequate support. While asserting that the welfare of the child must always remain the paramount concern of professionals working with such families, it argues that there is often scope for professional responses to parental substance misuse and mental health issues to be more effective in supporting parents to safeguard the welfare of their children.

This chapter provides definitions of key terms and concepts used in this book and statistics to indicate the numbers of children and families affected. It gives a broad outline of the policy and legislative context, highlighting the continuing difficulties with achieving the necessary coordination of policies and services to effect a 'whole-family approach'. The importance of the parenting role in many adult lives and the likely impact of parental mental health/substance misuse problems on children in such families are too often overlooked by agencies whose primary focus is on the individual adult client.

Underpinning principles

Most parents, including those who have substance misuse and/or mental health difficulties, are deeply concerned for the welfare of their children. Many parents in these circumstances, given the right support, are nonetheless able to parent their children well. However, when parents lack the personal resources or external support required to meet their children's needs, their children suffer. It is therefore essential that practitioners – in all relevant fields – do not lose sight of children's needs and act in a timely and appropriate manner in order to meet them.

The interests of the child and their right to be protected from harm are always paramount. In addition to this, though, there is often much that can and should be done to support parenting and safeguard children. Such support can prevent parents' problems escalating to a point where the removal of the child from their parents' care becomes unavoidable. At all stages, professionals should be asking: Given that this is the situation, what are the needs of this child? What are the immediate and longer-term risks to this child? What things can be done that will minimise the impact of this on the child? And what might make a difference to how well the parents can meet or understand the needs and experiences of their child? Can these changes be achieved within a timeframe that will meet the child's needs?

Central to this handbook and the original Building Resilience project from which the original ideas were drawn, is a belief that more often than not there is scope for practitioner responses to parental substance misuse and mental health problems to be more effective in supporting parenting and, in turn, the welfare of children. Stigmatisation of such parents is a major factor in both worsening their circumstances and in reducing the likelihood of them feeling able to access or ask for support. An increased awareness of stigma and of negative assumptions that can compound parents' difficulties can lead to more thorough, open explorations of their needs and potential.

Also, an increased understanding among relevant practitioners of what factors are likely to enhance the resilience of children and their families would enable them to respond more confidently and proactively to family difficulties.

This handbook then is about supporting families with substance misuse or mental health problems, or both, and enabling parents and their children to cope better with their circumstances. It explores and shares information that might help practitioners to harness the strengths, positive motivation and values of many adults. There will inevitably be times when there is a tension between the needs of children and the priorities and capacities of their parents. In these circumstances it will sometimes, regrettably, be necessary for children to be removed from the care of their parents. However, this need can be averted in some cases if professional knowledge and skills are enhanced to enable services to work more preventively and proactively with parents. Early intervention and support for families can be effective in keeping them together, safeguarding children and helping parents to support their child's well-being.

Definitions
Resilience

> A universal capacity that allows a person, group or community to prevent, minimise or overcome the damaging effects of adversity. (Grotberg 1997, p.7 in Newman and Blackburn 2002)

Certain factors (often referred to as 'protective factors'), such as the presence of an unconditionally supportive adult from either within the family or external to it, have been seen in a number of studies to play an important part in minimising the impact of family problems on children. The presence of such factors can be seen as leading to better outcomes for children. Resilience factors are discussed further in Chapter 3.

Mental health problems

This handbook focuses specifically on circumstances where parents or their children are experiencing problems and these are linked to a parent's mental health. This will include minor mental health problems, such as a one-off or occasional period of depression or anxiety, through to the most severe disorders, such as bipolar disorder or schizophrenia. However, minor problems are only included if it can be said of the parents experiencing them that they are:

> experiencing such emotional distress that they find it hard to function as well as they would wish, and they and/or others are concerned about the actual or likely impact this is having on their children. (Tunnard 2004, p.7)

Some studies referred to within this handbook may use the term 'mental illness' instead. Where this is used, the following definition may be useful:

> A term used by doctors and other health professionals to describe clinically recognisable patterns of psychological symptoms or behaviour causing acute or chronic ill-health, personal distress or distress to others. (World Health Organization 1992)

For definitions of specific categories of mental health diagnoses, Falkov (1998, pp.37–55) provides summaries; and some of the mental-health related websites listed in the Further Resources section of this handbook provide useful information.

Substance misuse

This term includes those using any substances, including alcohol, prescribed medication or illegal drugs. 'Misuse' rather than 'use' is referred to in order to distinguish between the recreational user and the dependent user whose behaviour, mood or other life circumstances are adversely affected by their use of the substance.

Another term that is often used in this handbook, particularly if referring to information from the *Hidden Harm* reports from the Advisory Council on the Misuse of Drugs (ACMD 2011), is problem drug use. The Advisory Council defines problem drug use as that which has:

> serious negative consequences of a physical, psychological, social and interpersonal, financial or legal nature for users and those around them. (ACMD 2011, P. 7)

Whilst much of the discussion about parental substance misuse will be general, occasionally alcohol misuse is referred to separately because it brings with it some distinct issues. Also, services are often set up separately for drug users and alcohol users within voluntary and statutory services.

For the classification of individual drugs and their effects, there are a number of useful summaries: FRANK[1], Kroll and Taylor (2003) and Hart and Powell (2006).

Coexisting/multiple needs and dual diagnosis

This is a term used to describe the presence in an individual of two or more categories of need from a range including, for example, learning disabilities, mental health issues and substance misuse issues. In this handbook, it is generally used to indicate the presence of mental health problems along with substance misuse issues, sometimes referred to as dual diagnosis.

Defining dual diagnosis can be contentious. Miller (1994) highlighted the key requirement of another disorder existing independent of an addictive disorder. Using this criterion raises the question as to how 'independent' substance misuse and mental health problems are from each other. For example, in some circumstances it can be argued that substance use has led to mental health difficulties or, conversely, that substance use is a form of 'self-medication' for emotional distress arising from mental health problems. Therefore an understanding of the mental health issues and the substance use, in addition to a consideration of the interaction between the two, is necessary.

Velleman (2004), Falkov (1998) and Cleaver, Unell and Aldgate (1999) found dual diagnosis to be associated with: reduced treatment compliance; more severe mental health problems; greater risks of self-harm and harm to others; greater family discord; an increased likelihood of domestic violence; and increased social and financial difficulties. Furthermore, the presence of coexisting parental mental health problems, parental substance misuse and/or domestic violence is now well known as increasing potential risks to children (Taylor 2013).

Whilst coexisting or multiple needs, for example parental substance misuse and parental mental health problems, together cause an increased professional concern (Forrester 2000), which is potentially compounded by services tending not to be geared up to meeting overlapping needs effectively, the interrelatedness of the mental health and substance use are only explored to a limited extent in this handbook.

---

1   www.talktofrank.com

Prevalence

Mental health problems and substance misuse are not readily measurable in terms of prevalence. Much of people's emotion and behaviour is unknowable and it is only when people are formally diagnosed or identified through services that individuals are included within prevalence figures. Secrecy – and the inevitability of this due to stigma and illegality (in the case of drug use) – further limits the chances of prevalence figures being accurate. It is likely therefore that the figures used by official bodies, such as the Advisory Council on the Misuse of Drugs, are underestimations. Also, mental health varies over time, with many people experiencing episodes of problems but feeling well in between. Similarly, substance use or misuse is a behaviour and even those who view addiction as a permanent illness that has to be managed would acknowledge that its impact, visibility and how it is seen and experienced by individuals changes over time. That said, the following figures that are available give some indication of prevalence.

Mental health problems

One in six adults experiences at least one period of minor mental health difficulty, such as depression or anxiety, in their lifetime (Social Exclusion Unit 2004) and at the time of their illness a quarter to a half of these will be parents. To emphasise the importance of the issue for all agencies and professionals, it is estimated that in a class of 26 primary school children, 6 or 7 will live with a mother with mental health problems (SCIE 2012). Prevalence is highest in women and lone parents (Meltzer, Gill and Petticrew 1995) and those in socially disadvantaged groups or communities. One in forty adults experience serious and enduring mental health problems in their lifetime, such as schizophrenia, severe depression, bipolar disorder or dual diagnosis (Tunnard 2004).

At least a quarter of adults known to mental health services are parents; a third of children known to adolescent mental health services have parents with a psychiatric disorder; and parental mental health problems or substance misuse is recorded in at least a third of families referred to social services due to child protection concerns (Falkov 1998) while a review of 40 serious case reviews found that almost two-thirds (60%) of children lived in a household with a parent or carer with current or past mental illness (Brandon *et al.* 2012).

Alcohol misuse

Although figures on prevalence vary for the reasons outlined previously, there is little argument with the fact that many children are living in families seriously affected by alcohol. It is estimated that approaching 300,000 children in the UK live with a harmful drinker (Manning *et al.* 2009) while according to unpublished National Treatment Agency (NTA) figures, some 53 per cent of adults in alcohol treatment are parents (Martins 2013). Children known to be living with parental alcohol misuse are thought to number between 780,000 and 1.3 million (Prime Minister's Strategy Unit 2003), which equates to 1 in 11 children living with problem drinkers (Turning Point 2006). Men are more likely to report hazardous drinking and signs of dependence than women (Office for National Statistics in Gopfert, Webster and Seeman 2004) and there has been a growth in problem drinking overall since the early 1990s.

Drug misuse

The number of adults known to have 'problem drug use' (as defined by the Advisory Council on the Misuse of Drugs) is growing, and the annual numbers of those accessing drug services doubled between 1996 and 2000. Conservative estimates are that between 200,000 and 300,000 children in England and Wales are affected by parental problem drug use. Many of these children will be living with other relatives and not with their parents – only a third of fathers and two-thirds of mothers with problem drug use are usually living with their children (ACMD 2003). At the same time, according to NTA figures over 50 per cent of people in drug treatment during 2011–2012 were either parents or lived with children (NTA 2012).

Parental substance misuse features strongly in child protection work (in 20–70% of social worker's caseloads), and 20–50 per cent of children subject to a child protection plan involve parental substance misuse (Martins 2013).

Coexisting/multiple needs

A high number of adults have both mental health and substance misuse difficulties. Morris and Wates (2006) report on studies that found such overlaps within groups of services' users. For example, one study found 75 per cent of drug service users and 85 per cent of alcohol service users had additional mental health problems, and 44 per cent of Community Mental Health Team users reported substance misuse or problem drinking within the previous 12 months.

Legislation and policy context

The legislative and policy background to service provision for families affected by parental mental health, substance misuse and child welfare issues is complex, with a raft of legal and policy measures that have been introduced at different times and for different reasons. The consequence of this can be a lack of clarity and a failure by legislators and service planners to make links between them.

It can be difficult to keep abreast of the policy and legislative context within one professional arena, for example within children's social care or adult mental health. It is all the more difficult to keep up with policy or legislation in other fields. The following areas of policy and legislation (though not exhaustive) are of particular relevance:

- cross-cutting policy and legislation
- children's and adults' social care
- health reforms

- welfare reform
- mental health
- drugs and alcohol
- families and parenting
- disability.

A summary of the above areas of policy and legislation (which highlights policy/legislative arena issues relevant to parenting and family welfare from each) can be found in the Appendix.

On the whole, legislation and policies that relate to mental health and to drugs tended, until fairly recently, to focus on the single adult user. They didn't place sufficient responsibilities and duties on the responding services to meet wider families' needs. In fact they often failed to acknowledge any overlap or tension between the rights and responsibilities of one member of the family (for example a parent) with those of another (for example a child or young carer). The 1995 10-year Drug Strategy (Home Office, Department of Health and Department for Education 1995), for example, focused on adult drug use as a criminal activity and did not acknowledge parenting as a feature of many drug users' lives and responsibilities. There was a tendency to focus on the consequences of parental drug use rather than on helping parents manage or change their use of drugs. More recently there have been attempts to redress this. For example, the 2008 strategy (HM Government 2008) paid much more attention to supporting drug users as parents. More recently, the coalition-government revised Drug Strategy (HM Government 2010) places an emphasis on preventing problems from arising, stresses the need for adults' and children's services to devise protocols for working together and states that drug and alcohol services should be represented on Local Safeguarding Children's Boards (LSCBs).

Whilst much of the legislation and policy aimed at children does broadly include addressing their needs in relation to any familial factors affecting them, the implementation of such policies tends to be seen as the domain of children's services and not (in practice) those whose primary clients are adults.

The Children Act 2004 sought to strengthen partnership working across agencies to promote children's well-being. Many of its provisions remain in place, including:

- a reciprocal duty among a list of partners to promote cooperation to improve the well-being of children (section 10)
- a duty on partners to safeguard and promote the welfare of children.

Whilst the separation of adults' and children's services has been largely supported through legislation, there has been recognition in guidance and policy of the importance of bridging these divides and more recently this imperative seems to be getting stronger.

The statutory guidance, *Working Together to Safeguard Children*, has been through a number of revisions, most recently in March 2015 (HM Government 2015). It emphasises two key principles: that safeguarding is everyone's responsibility and that services should be based on the needs and views of children. It continues to highlight the role of all professionals, including those supporting adults with children, to identify problems and secure help early for those children and families that need it. The Care and Support (Eligibility Criteria) Regulations 2014 accompanying the Care Act 2014 set out the eligibility threshold for adults with care and support needs. The threshold is based on identifying how a person's needs affect a range of outcomes and their well-being, and amongst the relevant outcomes is that of the adult's ability to carry out parenting responsibilities.

Another key piece of legislation is the Children and Families Act 2014, which includes amendments to the Children Act 1989, setting out duties of local authorities to young carers. There is further support for this within the Care and Support statutory guidance, which complements and explains the Care Act and related regulations. It makes clear that children should not undertake inappropriate or excessive caring roles and once the local authority has identified a young carer requires them to undertake an assessment of their needs.

To conclude, although the legislation and policy have not consistently acknowledged 'parenting' and the links between children and adults (in relation to services, needs, rights and responsibilities), increasingly provisions are being included within the legislation and guidance and some drivers put in place to try to address this.

While the differences are manifold there are a number of similarities in the issues facing adults' and children's services, including the tension between high eligibility thresholds and the vision of providing preventative services. The current drive towards more joint commissioning, a greater 'outcomes focus', needs analysis and more multi-agency working, is positive. However, it is essential that at a local level, opportunities are not lost for adults' and children's services to become more directly connected, because:

> in a system that 'thinks family' contact with any service offers an open door into a broader system of joined up support… Front-line staff are alert to wider individual and family risk factors, and practitioners consider the causes and wider impacts of presenting problems. (Cabinet Office and Social Exclusion Taskforce 2008, p.4)

The service context

The impact of both parental mental health issues and substance misuse on the work of relevant services is 'pervasive, hidden and under recognised' (Kearney *et al.* 2003a, p.7), with a lack of information systems in place to capture the size of the problem. Despite the lack of official statistics on parental mental health issues, it has been estimated that up to 30 per cent of the adults in contact with specialised mental health services have dependent children (Melzer 2008).

The organisation of services aimed at supporting such families (or the individuals within them) is complicated and disparate. A complex range of advice, assessment and treatment services are available to varying extents in local areas. Services struggle to work together in a coordinated way. Problems for families in accessing appropriate support are therefore common. Resource constraints (and the resulting high eligibility thresholds) within health and social care services mean tight gatekeeping and responses that tend to be reactive and crisis-led.

The Department for Education (DfE, formerly DCSF) wants those who most need parental and family support to be able to access well-coordinated, high-quality support early enough so as to reduce the number of vulnerable families who go on to develop complex problems in the future. The department's earlier analysis (Department for Education and Skills 2006a) confirming a gap between this desired state and the market highlighted a focus by the statutory sector on remedial interventions with minimal resources for prevention, and it suggested that this makes it unlikely that ongoing support was available for as long as parents needed it and that fathers and black and minority ethnic groups in particular were not being engaged with effectively, especially at the lower tiers of need.

More recent high-profile government reviews such as the Munro review (Department for Education 2011) and the Graham Allen review (HM Government 2011) both placed emphasis on early support for children and families. Also, although the coalition government's Early Intervention Grant has represented a continuing fall in spending for non-ring-fenced services, in its advice to local areas the government has emphasised targeting support to families with multiple needs and the most vulnerable families.

In a similar vein, initiatives such as the coalition's Troubled Families programme have continued this focus. Launched in 2010 with £450 million to tackle the difficulties posed by those branded the most 'troubled' 120,000 families, the programme was expanded for a further five years from 2015/16 to reach up to an additional 400,000 families across England with a further commitment of £200 million to fund the first year. Local authorities have been exhorted to join up local services, deal with problems on a whole-family rather than individual level and appoint a keyworker to families. Of particular significance to the concerns of this handbook is the fact that from 2015, the expanded programme will also address families' mental and physical health needs including substance misuse.

Local areas, in responding to these reviews and initiatives have sought to establish Early Help services. While the models, structures and specific approaches used within these vary, they generally reflect attempts to create services that are more multi-agency, coordinated across service areas and accessible to children and families with multiple needs.

Additionally, some areas have been able to secure support for service and practice developments for families with multiple and complex needs through the government's Social Care Innovation programme, launched in October 2013. Successful applicants include Hertfordshire, which has chosen to focus its programme on 'the most vulnerable families' in the county. The programme will see the establishment of Family Safeguarding teams across the county, which alongside children's social workers will include domestic abuse specialists and community psychiatric nurses to focus on parental mental health and parental substance misuse. Like a number of other areas, Hertfordshire's programme also includes training in Motivational Interviewing (MI), an attempt to up-skill staff to improve engagement with families.

The backdrop to these developments is bleak, insofar as outcomes for children and the experiences of children and adults within such families is concerned. The outcomes for children in families where there is parental 'problem drug use' are known to be poor, with less than half of all problem drug-using parents in the UK living with their children (Gruer and Ainsworth 2003). Mostly, their children end up living with other relatives and 9 per cent become looked after under the Children Act 1989.

In their research into parental substance misuse and child welfare in social services, Forrester and Harwin (2006) found a third of cases in overall social work caseloads (in four London boroughs) had substance misuse issues noted. They found, despite substance use being so prevalent among caseloads, that social workers were poorly prepared for working with these issues. Two years after they first looked at case files:

- 54 per cent of the children no longer lived at home
- a third had been removed by care proceedings
- the majority lived with kinship carers, with or without a court order attached
- 8 per cent were adopted
- 16 per cent were in short-term foster care.

In relation to violence in the home and in relation to alcohol use (particularly when these occurred together) overall, Forrester and Harwin's (2006) research pointed to a tendency for under-intervention. If children in such families were removed from home this happened much later when they were older, even though in the sample the overall outcomes were worse for those who remained at home. Velleman (2004) similarly found that drug-misusing parents were more likely to be rated high risk and to have their children removed than alcohol-misusing parents. This could be in part due to: a higher level of familiarity by workers with alcohol; the illegality or stigmatisation of substance misuse; and a lack of recognition of the potential long-term impact on children of exposure to parental alcohol misuse.

It is still the case that whilst intervention is occurring, it is occurring at the 'heavy end' of family difficulty – too late and with the child protection process and legal intervention all too often being seen as the only realistic response by that stage. For children of alcohol-misusing parents, intervention is occurring even later. A lack of preventative services seems to be linked to: high eligibility criteria; a lack of understanding about how to intervene constructively with families; and a reluctance by families to ask for help for fear their children will be removed.

The picture is similarly bleak in relation to responses to parental mental health difficulty. Thresholds for intervention, and in particular for specialist services, are so high that they are not accessible for families assessed as having anything less than 'severe' or 'acute' need (Tunnard 2004). It is very difficult for families with mild or moderate mental health issues to access preventative support (from statutory services) in relation to their mental health needs, even though the impact on their children could be felt to be 'severe'.

As far as possible, services aim to support adults with mental health problems to remain in the home with support, but this can only be beneficial if the interrelated needs of other family members in the home are considered appropriately. Tunnard (2004) reported that there was a lack of appropriate services provided to parents with mental health difficulties, with a significant number receiving no outside help. Of those who did receive help, many found it intrusive and of poor quality.

When it is necessary for parents with mental health problems to be hospitalised, this can be traumatic for them and their family members. Psychiatric wards can be potentially frightening places for children and do not provide privacy or a suitable environment for parents and their children to have positive contact. There is a lack of family-friendly facilities, although there are some examples of family rooms being set up, such as the one at Stoddart House in Aintree (arising from Barnardo's Keeping the Family in Mind project collaboration with Mersey Care. See the 'Training and development resources' section in the Further Resources section).

Also, as a result of resource constraints mental health care is often inadequate, both within the community and for inpatients. For example, while access to some approaches such as cognitive behavioural therapy is helping some service users, overall access to talking therapies is lacking due to long waiting lists, financial constraints and a lack of therapists.

To conclude, definitions and prevalence of parental mental health and parental substance misuse are imprecise, while the policy, legislation and service context can be fragmented and complex. Nonetheless, considerable amounts of data and research together with legislative and policy drivers are now available to practitioners and managers to support their efforts to develop more coherent and connected services to address better the needs of affected children and adults.

2
The potential impact on children and families

This chapter gives an overview of key research findings on the risks and impacts of parental substance misuse and mental health problems on children. Findings indicate that these parental problems are usually of great significance to children in affected families. Possible adverse impacts are outlined in terms of the three domains of the *Framework for the Assessment of Children in Need and their Families: Family and Environmental Factors, Parenting Capacity and Children's Developmental Needs* (Department of Health 2000).

It stresses that assessing such impacts on individual children and families requires analysis, reflection and self-awareness in those undertaking it. A clear focus on questioning and exploring the everyday experience of family members is needed – rather than focusing primarily or exclusively on crisis or 'unusual' incidents – along with a child-focused, ecological approach and knowledge of research and other evidence about effective interventions.

This chapter provides an essential overview of some of the research available on the potential implications for children and families when parental substance misuse or parental mental health problems are present, to increase the awareness that relevant practitioners and professionals have of these issues. This awareness should be utilised in tandem with an understanding of resilience factors (discussed in Chapter 3) and approaches to support (discussed in Chapter 5) that might help alleviate or reduce negative impacts.

Parents who misuse substances, and those with mental health difficulties, are obviously not homogeneous groups and there will be significant diversity of experience. However, from what is known, it is evident that parental substance misuse and parental mental health problems are usually of great significance to the welfare of families. Literature and research relating to parenting in these circumstances have pointed to a range of common experiences such as: stigma and discrimination; poverty; isolation; a potential inconsistency of care; and disruptions and crises. These parental issues can be seen to have long-lasting effects on outcomes for children, potentially into adulthood. For example, an estimated third to two-thirds of children whose parents have mental health problems will experience mental health difficulties themselves (SCIE 2012). The physical effects of substance misuse on unborn or new-born babies can be long lasting (Barnard and Barlow 2003) and young people exposed to a culture of substance misuse may continue this on into their own adulthood (Martins 2013).

Whilst by no means always the case, the risks posed by parental substance misuse and parental mental health problems can be extremely serious or even fatal. Parental substance misuse significantly increases the risk of physical and emotional neglect and in some cases substance misuse is a key factor in a child's death or serious injury (through ingesting methadone or exposure to serious risks such as scalding due to lack of supervision).

Whilst most parents with mental health difficulties don't pose a risk of child abuse to their children, risks are heightened if their difficulties are psychotic in nature or are coupled with substance misuse. An increased risk of maltreatment by mothers with severe depression and those with schizophrenia who draw their children into their negative delusions has also been long established (Falkov 1998). Even where parents don't pose a physical risk to their children, there is a possibility of children being frightened by severe mood changes or bizarre or unusual behaviours when their parents are unwell. In all cases, the risk of difficulties escalating and the levels of unmet need or risk increasing are compounded by a lack of appropriate responses from services.

Both parental substance misuse and parental mental health problems are known to be frequent key factors in cases where children have been seriously injured or have died. In the 2012 biennial analysis of serious case reviews, parental mental ill health was found to be a factor in 60 per cent of serious case reviews and parental substance misuse was present in 42 per cent (Brandon *et al.* 2012). It has also become increasingly well known that parental problems such as mental ill health, substance misuse and/or domestic abuse often coexist, occurring together in the same family, and that the presence of one, two or all three of these issues is a common characteristic in situations leading to serious case reviews. In their 2012 review, Brandon *et al.* found at least one of these characteristics to be present in 86 per cent of cases, all three together in 20 per cent and that it was 'more common for these features to exist in combination than singly' (p.37). It stands to reason and is well recognised that when these issues occur together, the risks to children are heightened (Martins 2013). Cleaver *et al.* (2011) in Taylor (2013) describe the combined nature of these dynamic factors as 'multiplicative' in impact. Therefore it is essential that in trying to understand the impact of these circumstances on children, the relationship between factors and the way in which difficulties accumulate or 'multiply' are considered. This is not easy to do but will be aided by a baseline understanding of some of the potential impacts that these issues can bring about individually.

Before setting out what the research tells us about impacts on children it is important to point out that there are a number of limitations with the literature and research. First, the majority of the literature and research that can potentially be drawn on comes from the USA, where the context (law, service structures and practice cultures) is often different. Furthermore, in much of the available research (particularly relating to parental mental health), 'parent' is often synonymous with 'mothers', with less consideration given to fathers and the impact on their relationship with their children. It is also important to note that of the research relating to parental mental health, the predominant focus is upon depression (Parrott, Jacobs and Roberts 2008). Furthermore, there is a lack of research into the perspective of children and young people regarding their experiences. Another important feature is that most of the attention focuses on identifying risks and poor outcomes that are often associated with such parental difficulties, rather than focusing on 'what goes well'. As the majority of studies are based on samples of parents who are known to services, the findings are likely to be skewed (Olsen and Wates 2003). There has been little research on how parents and children fare when given appropriate and timely support. That said, the information that is available is useful if viewed in context and applied critically with a focus towards families' individual circumstances.

For additional information see the useful overviews of research that have been done by Cleaver, Unell, and Aldgate (1999, 2011), Tunnard (2002a, 2002b, 2004), Kroll and Taylor (2003), Parrott *et al.* 2008 and Taylor (2013), which are drawn on in this summary.

Below is an exploration of some of the issues known to be frequently associated with these circumstances. The three domains of the *Framework for the Assessment of Children in Need and their Families* (Department of Health 2000) and of the *Common Assessment Framework* (HM Government 2006) – family and environmental factors, parenting capacity and the child's developmental needs – have been used as headings for ease of reference. For those who are not familiar with the three domains they are based on the assessment triangle (Figure 2.1), which forms the basis for assessments undertaken by children and family social workers in conjunction with other relevant practitioners and professionals. This 'ecological' approach is based on the premise that the well-being of a family can best be understood if there is an appreciation of the ways in which the children's developmental needs, parents' capacity to respond to those needs, and wider environmental factors interact with one another over time (NSPCC 2000).

Figure 2.1: Assessment triangle

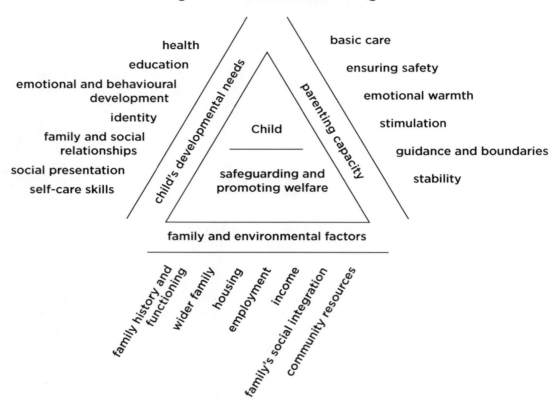

Adapted from Hart and Powell 2006 (p.28)

Family and environmental factors

Anecdotal evidence and inspections have highlighted that 'family and environmental factors' is often the 'missing side of the triangle' within assessments (Jack and Gill 2003) because not enough attention is paid to considering the wider social and environmental factors that affect families and, in turn, parenting. One reason could be that factors such as poverty and deprivation are hard to influence at the practitioner or indeed local services level. Such issues therefore come to be seen as too difficult, residual or less relevant to the 'task' of assessing needs of individual children and families. However, understanding and acknowledging the context of a family's experience is essential to good assessment practice, and service users are likely to be more engaged with services when their whole experience is recognised and attention is paid to the challenges they genuinely face in their lives, which originate both within their internal and external world (Kroll and Taylor 2003).

Family history and functioning

Previous experience of parents

Many adults with substance misuse and/or mental health problems have experienced adversity in their own childhoods. Exploring parents' experiences of being parented, along with establishing how family members experience each other in the present day, can lead to useful insights. Mental health issues may well be triggered by previous experiences or exacerbated by the ways in which the family functions in the present day (such as a culture of secrecy or 'not complaining') and substance misuse may be a way of avoiding or being distracted from other problems (Bennett 1989).

Support of partner

Whether one or both parents or carers are experiencing mental ill health or misusing substances may significantly affect the impact on the child. Where only one parent has mental health problems or substance misuse issues, their partner can play a key role in minimising the negative impact on children. In relation to substance misuse, studies have highlighted the benefit to children of stable relationships.

Where mothers have agreed that they wanted and planned to reduce their substance use, their partner's support of that decision was 'the most effective influence for positive change' (Tunnard 2002a, p.25). However, a partner's own substance use was cited as the most negative influence (Tunnard 2002a). Much of the research about this is specific to mothers with mental health or substance misuse issues, although it seems likely to apply to both sexes.

'Partner difficulties' have been found to be a common and contributory source of stress to parents with mental health problems who are in touch with statutory services and this is especially the case for depressed mothers (Tunnard 2004). Conversely, supportive fathers can 'buffer' children from a range of difficulties, including, but not limited to, maternal depression, and where fathers are perceived as supportive, new mothers 'experience less postpartum distress' (Fatherhood Institute 2013).

Separations and changes

Children are at an increased likelihood of experiencing separations, which may be short or long term, including, for example, planned or emergency hospitalisation or treatment for parents. Sometimes separations are a result of children being removed from their parents' care for periods of respite in order to prevent or address a crisis situation in which the child or parent's needs would be compromised if they remained at home.

Children may experience a number of minor or major changes in their family, including in the roles that family members take on. For example, a 'well parent' may perform tasks and essentially step into the role normally held by the parent with mental health problems (Falkov 1998). Such changes can be unsettling and are sometimes resisted by children.

Family conflict

There are significant associations between both mental health problems and substance misuse and domestic violence. Excessive alcohol use is also frequently associated with violence in families (McCarthy and Galvani 2010). Hamilton and Collins (1981) and Powers (1986) found 80 per cent of spouse-to-spouse violence to be alcohol related. It is difficult to untangle the interrelationship between substance use, mental health and family discord or violence. Hester, Pearson and Harwin (2003) stress that substance use can be seen in some cases as a response to domestic violence; and a consideration of such issues is important within assessments and dialogues with those affected.

Where conflict and domestic violence occur, outcomes for children worsen. As Galvani (2010) puts it, where children are exposed to both parental alcohol misuse and domestic abuse they are subject to 'a double dose of harm' (p.4). Furthermore, if arguments involve the child (in reality or in the child's perception) the negative impact on children is increased further (Velleman 1993).

Wider family

Given the potential for separations, change and parental conflict, the role of other relatives is significant, and extended family members often provide considerable support. However, parents with mental health problems can experience difficulties in maintaining positive relationships with wider family members, often due to stigma and when their behaviour results in disapproval or misunderstandings. Where the support of wider family or friends is available to families under stress, this is valued and becomes most crucial in times of crisis. Relatives are likely to need support and information to help them understand the needs and issues facing the parent (Tunnard 2004; NHS England and NHS Improving Quality 2014).

In the case of substance-misusing mothers, many report positive relationships with their mother or another female relative (Tunnard 2002a). However, in some cases, relationships with relatives may have broken down previously, due to the rejection of the parent because of their substance misuse or the secrecy surrounding it (Kroll and Taylor 2003), and in such instances this proves a significant barrier to familial support being provided by the wider family.

Housing

There are higher rates of depression among the populations of deprived areas than in more affluent areas. Unsafe neighbourhoods, poor housing, overcrowding and disputes with neighbours all increase stress significantly and are more commonly experienced by depressed mothers than other mothers (Tunnard 2004). This is compounded further for black and minority ethnic families who additionally often experience racism and discrimination (Social Exclusion Unit 2004) within local areas.

For families affected by substance misuse, in many cases the financial demands of securing drugs on a daily basis can lead to a lack of furniture and unpaid bills, resulting in erratic supplies of utilities such as gas, electricity and telephone access.

Sometimes failures to pay rent or mortgages lead to eviction and a succession of short-term unsuitable housing (Cleaver *et al.* 1999).

Employment

Research by Gould (2006) indicates less than a quarter of adults with long-term mental health problems are employed and that many of those in employment have periods of absence affecting their income and career prospects. The Social Exclusion Unit highlights the tendency for adults with mental health problems to experience discrimination by potential employers and for black and minority ethnic adults to experience additional discrimination on the grounds of both their health status and ethnicity when seeking work (Social Exclusion Unit 2004). In fact, long working hours and/or a loss of control at work can potentially trigger parental mental health problems (Parrott *et al.* 2008), thus indicating the potential for multiple stresses and a 'vicious circle'.

The unpredictable and inconsistent effect of drug or alcohol use on individuals can make it hard to sustain employment. Once people are out of employment, studies in Europe and USA have shown this to be negatively correlated with drinking (particularly binge drinking), which is at increased likelihood of occurring (ICAP 2011).

Income

People with mental health problems or substance misuse issues have an increased likelihood of being affected by poverty and having low incomes. Sustained use, for example, of heroin or cocaine can be very expensive and diminish family resources. The link between poverty and drug use is complex but, overall, substance misuse is often strongly associated with poverty (Martins 2013) and drug users tend to be found in higher numbers in socially deprived areas. People with mental health problems tend to be on low incomes (exacerbated by employment issues). This creates stress and in turn often compounds mental health problems as well as increasing the risk of substance misuse and relapse (Fraser *et al.* 2006).

Family's social integration

There is increased likelihood of children in these circumstances experiencing isolation from a wider network of social support (Martins 2013). This is in part due to the stigma and secrecy that often surround mental health and substance misuse issues, in addition to the social exclusion that results from poverty and deprivation. These difficulties are compounded further for some groups such as lone parent families and for black and minority ethnic families. Isolated parents have fewer opportunities to get support from other parents; and their children are less likely to have friends visit them at home. Whilst Velleman and Orford (1999) did not find such isolation in problem-drinking families, they did find a knock-on effect on children's friendships. Often they were embarrassed by their homes and had a sense of 'being apart' from others.

When there is parental substance misuse, in some cases friends of the parent/family offer considerable support, whereas in others friends and associates who are also involved in substance misuse can pose additional risks that are 'sometimes as difficult to control as the drug use itself' (Tunnard 2002a).

Community resources

A tendency for families to 'close in on themselves' due to social isolation is exacerbated by poor or stigmatising community resources and a fear of being judged as not coping or being a poor parent. With substance misuse this can result in families retreating further into a substance-using environment to the exclusion of wider support (Velleman 1993). This worsens further when there are specific cultural issues and increased stigma regarding drug or alcohol use (Patel 2000; Tunnard 2002a). Where families are affected by mental health issues, a tendency towards increased isolation due to stigma, poverty or wariness of services and of others significantly increases vulnerability.

The availability of good community resources is an important factor affecting the level of adverse impact on families (Kroll and Taylor 2003). High-quality and accessible childcare, health care, transport, leisure and educational facilities can all make a big difference to how isolated or supported families are.

Community resources that provide a range of services within one location can be particularly useful. For pregnant drug users, for example, uptake of appointments within clinics is likely to be improved by the provision of accessible, multidisciplinary support in one location, given the often chaotic lifestyles associated with drug use and the other barriers caused by social deprivation.

Parenting capacity

It is important to reiterate that many people with mental health difficulties and/or who use drugs do manage to care adequately for their children. However, many experience difficulties at some time or other in managing to meet their children's needs. If those with difficulties are insufficiently supported or the difficulties are too severe, it can result in children facing greater stresses and risks and experiencing poorer outcomes.

Basic care

In parents affected by mental health problems or substance misuse, a lack of energy, alertness or motivation can – and often does – affect the likelihood of basic care and chores being performed consistently. This can affect activities such as maintaining bath and bedtime routines, regular mealtimes, household chores and hygiene, and getting children to school on time.

In her review of the literature and research, Tunnard (2002b) found that the likelihood of children being at risk of neglect tends to increase if parents are affected by mental health problems or substance misuse. Forrester (2000) found in a localised study that over 60 per cent of children on the child protection register for neglect (and emotional abuse) had one or more substance-misusing parents. It is often the case that deficits in children's care may be deemed individually as low-level concerns. But over time, neglect of children's physical care needs can be chronic and their impact enduring, not least if their health is affected or their hygiene, which can impact on self-esteem and relationships with others.

Ensuring safety

Substance misuse can lead to drowsiness and a lack of physical coordination, increasing the risk of parental accidents, including dropping a baby or child, decreased awareness of environmental risks and lower levels of supervision, which can lead to accidents for children. There are additional risks if drug paraphernalia such as needles and lighters are left where children can reach them. Storing methadone (or other drugs) where children can access them can cause immediate and serious dangers to children and can be fatal.

The preoccupation that can come with dependence and withdrawal, due to drug use, is likely to lead to a poorer awareness of children's needs and a reduced sensitivity to risk (Bates, Buchanan and Corby 1999). Similarly, mental health problems, depression or intrusive thoughts and the effects of medication may reduce awareness of risks to children.

Emotional warmth

Parents can exhibit 'emotional unavailability' at particular times, for example when they are particularly unwell, preoccupied, on medication or using or withdrawing from drugs or alcohol. This can adversely affect children's identity, self-esteem and attachments.

'Low-warmth' and 'high-criticism' environments are associated with poorer outcomes for children. Such environments are prevalent where there is parental alcohol misuse and some problem drug use (Kroll and Taylor 2003; Brisby, Baker and Hedderwick 1997), including amphetamine use, which can be associated with parental irritability and aggression (Tunnard 2002a).

Stimulation

Around 10 to 15 per cent of women are affected by a heightened risk of depression after childbirth (Falkov 1998) and are likely to spend less time touching and looking at their baby. Where postnatal depression or maternal depression continues, a lower quality of interaction is found in the child's second year and insecure attachment is more likely to become apparent in the child's third year (Tunnard 2004).

More generally, when parents become emotionally less available to their children (as a result of low mood, effects of medication or substance misuse or due to substance withdrawal) this can result in a lack of stimulation and, in turn, disrupted attachments.

Guidance and boundaries

In the case of parental mental ill health, the effects of medication or the 'absent mindedness' or internal preoccupation that can accompany distress or depression can reduce parents' ability to supervise or set boundaries for their children.

Conversely, parents experiencing delusions, paranoia or anxiety may be excessively concerned about real or imagined risks to their child, causing them to set over-rigid boundaries or to restrict freedom or opportunities for their child.

As children become older, the problems arising from a lack of consistency, for example behavioural problems, can become more pronounced. Brisby *et al.* (1997) found there was often an authoritarian parenting style in problem-drinking families, but that periods of inebriation could lead at other times to a more lax approach and indifference, which can be confusing and create unclear boundaries and insecurity for children.

Stability

Unpredictability within daily life is a feature for many children with parents with either mental health or substance misuse issues. In the case of substance misuse, if a parent's moods and the events of the day are dependent on whether and how they secure and take drugs, the child's world must seem a very unstable one. There is likely to be a lack of routine, structure and consistency, all of which are important factors for children's senses of security, confidence and boundaries. Planned family occasions or events may not happen and can cause worry and uncertainty (Brisby *et al.* 1997). For children this can lead to disappointment or a lack of positive experiences to draw from or look forward to. Rituals, defined by Velleman (2004, p.186) as 'repeated gathering or set modes of behaviour which define the occasion or the day as being special', are intended to cement family relationships. Alcohol or drug use can cause disruption to such occasions, as can parental mental health difficulties.

Children's developmental needs
Health

In families affected by parental substance misuse, the knock-on effects of poverty, poor diet, potential neglect and poor hygiene can have an adverse impact on children's health. This can be compounded if money that would otherwise be spent on children is diverted to drugs.

Children of substance-misusing parents may also exhibit psychosomatic responses to anxiety such as headaches, bedwetting and stomach aches (Kroll and Taylor 2003). Also, some health problems may not be picked up by school medical services due to absenteeism (Cleaver *et al.* 1999). Similarly, parents in these circumstances may be less likely to seek medical attention for sick children due to a fear of their circumstances being discovered (Cleaver *et al.* 2011).

In addition to the above issues, where babies are born with withdrawal symptoms the difficulties they experience with sleep, feeding, breathing and 'high-pitched crying' can make them hard to care for (Taylor 2013), which in turn may increase their risk of experiencing maltreatment (Kroll and Taylor 2003).

Young people whose parents misuse drugs are at increased risk of developing their own substance problems, which in turn adversely impact on their health. Overall, there is a lack of longitudinal studies regarding the impact of substance-misusing parents on the emotional and mental health of children and young people.

In her overview of mental health research, Tunnard (2004) reported that in the UK, children whose parents screened positive on a mental health questionnaire were three times more likely than others to have mental health problems themselves. As with substance misuse, there is a lack of longitudinal data in the UK concerning the impact of parental mental health problems on children's health. Some qualitative studies show children and young people of parents with mental health problems to be likely to experience increased anxiety, depression and fear of not being able to cope with life, and physical symptoms such as asthma, epilepsy and hair and weight loss. The increased mental health risk could be due to: genetic factors; feeling isolated or rejected as a child (including by the well parent if their attention was more focused on the unwell parent than the child); or learnt behaviour.

Pre- and post-birth issues

During pregnancy, substance-misusing women are less likely to access services and are more likely to neglect their own health and diet, which in turn affects their mental and physical preparation for the baby and the baby's health.

There is a great deal of research to indicate that alcohol and drug use can adversely impact the health and development of babies, particularly within the first 12 weeks of pregnancy (Cleaver, Unell and Aldgate 2011; Forrester 2012; Hepburn 2007 in Taylor 2013). The effect on babies of different drugs used by their mothers in pregnancy is variable and multiple drug use complicates this further. In addition to the potential for miscarriages, low birth weights, premature births and smaller head circumference, there is an increased risk of 'cot death' or Sudden Infant Death Syndrome (Forrester 2012). Complications brought about by drug use in pregnancy can potentially be fundamental and long lasting. They can include: developmental delay; obstetric complications; muscular twitching; irritability; poor concentration; feeding difficulties; high-pitched crying; and reduced responsiveness. Bonding can also be adversely affected (Taylor 2013). Where mothers have HIV or hepatitis B or C (risks associated with using contaminated drug paraphernalia) there is also the risk of transmission of this to the child. These risks can be reduced by immunisation, drug treatment and/or caesarean section. The issue of detoxification in pregnancy is particularly complex. For example the use of methadone can potentially adversely impact on the baby's health, but the sudden cessation of drugs can also carry risks. Therefore medical supervision is very important in order for careful assessment and analysis of individual needs and circumstances to take place. There is a need for continued research to inform practice, but the weight of evidence and opinion suggests that, in pregnancy, maintaining methadone or 'stable' drug use may be preferable to detoxification. (Forrester 2012; Cleaver *et al.* 2011 in Taylor 2013).

After the baby is born, if they have become physically dependent on opiates symptoms generally develop within between one and three days. They may experience withdrawal symptoms and some short-term effects such as gastrointestinal problems and poor weight gain. The research is less clear about long-term outcomes currently, although there are indications of a possible link with vision problems (Forrester 2012 in Taylor 2013) and cognitive problems in young children. In relation to cocaine use, some links are suggested to problems in attention and concentration 'although the role of environmental enrichment plays a critical role in reducing these' (Rayns *et al.* 2011 in Taylor 2013, p.6).

It is not just the drugs perceived as most harmful that present a potential risk to unborn babies. For example cannabis use generally involves smoking nicotine – frequently unfiltered – which in itself is seen as high risk in pregnancy (Forrester 2012 in Taylor 2013).

In the case of alcohol, broadly, the more volume consumed the greater the likely impact it will have, but it is also the case that regular moderate use can be less harmful than binge drinking (Hepburn 2007 in Taylor 2013). Forrester (2012) and Rayns *et al.* (2013) argue that alcohol is potentially the most harmful substance in relation to its impact due to the way it affects 'brain development at a critical time in the evolving foetal central nervous system' (Taylor 2013). The collection of potential symptoms that can arise from alcohol use in pregnancy, such as impaired growth, physical and cognitive developmental delays or abnormalities, behavioural difficulties and in some cases, distinctive facial or physical characteristics are broadly termed Foetal Alcohol Spectrum Disorder (FASD) of which there are different types including the most commonly known and severe, Foetal Alcohol Syndrome (Rayns *et al.* 2013).

Adult mental health problems can be exacerbated by, or even occur as a result of, pregnancy and childbirth and in turn have an impact on the child. Postnatal depression and the more serious condition postpartum psychosis affect, respectively, 10–15 per cent of mothers and two in every thousand mothers. Evidence shows an association between postnatal depression and problematic mother–infant relationships, with potential for adverse cognitive and emotional impacts on the developing child. Postpartum psychosis can carry greater risks of suicidal or infanticidal thoughts, hallucinations and delusions (Falkov 1998), though this is rare.

Education

The effect on routines and daily life of parental substance misuse or mental health problems can lead to erratic school attendance or difficulties with punctuality for many children. Children affected by chronic parental substance misuse are at increased likelihood of having difficulties with learning, reading and concentrating, thus affecting attainment (Cleaver *et al.* 2011; Taylor 2013). The anxiety that many children feel about their parents affects their ability to concentrate whilst in school. Some children leave early for this reason or phone parents during the day to check up on them. In the case of parental mental ill health, children have reported fearing that their parents will seriously harm themselves or attempt suicide whilst they are at school (Aldridge and Becker 2003). It is worth noting here that a third of children and young people classed as young carers look after a parent with mental health problems although they are the group least likely to be offered a carers assessment (SCIE 2010).

For some children, school can be a great source of stability and distraction from their problems at home and many do very well at school (Frank 1995) and view it as a haven. Parents also appear to think school is important and children generally agree with this (Tunnard 2002a). However, where children and young people take on a caring role within their family, due to parental mental health problems for example, this can reduce their academic achievement and formal and informal contact with school and friends, increasing their isolation. Also, some children do express a reluctance to confide in teachers and others who may be a potential source of support, as they fear poor responses from schools, including their privacy being compromised.

Emotional and behavioural development

Both parental mental health problems and parental substance misuse are associated with behavioural and mental health problems in children and young people. Taylor (2013) comments that perhaps the main impact on children and young people affected by parental substance misuse is a feeling of not coming first (in relation to the drugs) or feeling 'unloved or unwanted' (p.8).

Parents experiencing mood changes, parents withdrawing from those around them (including children) or the discord (or exaggerated intimacy) that can be associated with parental substance misuse or mental health problems can lead to children feeling fear, confusion or a sense of being in some way responsible. This can lead to behavioural difficulties or internalised emotional responses that are not readily observed or easily recognised. Also, where children feel worthless, powerless or hopeless about their situation or future this increases their vulnerability to negative peer-group pressure and self-destructive or even suicidal behaviour (Cleaver *et al.* 2011).

In relation to children living with schizophrenic parents specifically, Somers (2006 in Parrot *et al.* 2008) found children to be at increased likelihood of experiencing psychiatric disturbance, fear and stress brought about by their parent's behaviour and the social isolation resulting from their situation. For children living with parental depression, it is possible that their experience of this may differ depending on whether their mother or father is depressed because of potential differences in how male and female parents respond to their depression. Spector (2006 in Parrot *et al.* 2008, p.4) suggests that fathers/male carers are more likely to socially withdrawal and to present as 'irritable and cynical'. However, Parrott *et al.* (2008) cite findings related to the impact of paternal depression that indicate little difference between children and young people living with depressed fathers (as children or later as adults) and their peers who are not in this situation. Where mothers have depression it has been suggested that this can adversely impact on the attachment and bonding between children and their fathers (Peisah *et al.* 2004 in Parrott *et al.* 2008).

Whether or not children or young people living with parental substance misuse or parental mental health problems undertake practical or emotional care of their parents, many often worry about parents to the exclusion of themselves. When asked how their parent's illness affected them, half the children in a study (reported by Tunnard 2004) referred only to concerns felt about their parent. Various studies have shown that children are more concerned about the issues relating to the emotional than the practical support of their parent.

If parental problems result in secrecy, for example about illegal drug use or criminal activities associated with it, where children hold information (which they often do even though sometimes their parents don't realise or acknowledge it), this can lead to children and young people feeling burdened and more separate from their friends and others from whom they must keep the secret. Furthermore, as Taylor (2013) points out, parental substance misuse can be perceived and adopted by children and young people as an (albeit unhelpful) model for problem-solving.

Outcomes tend to be better when bad times are interspersed with good times in which children feel loved and well cared for. When negative experiences accumulate, or confused and inconsistent messages and care bring a sense of not being loved, impacts on children are worse (Kroll and Taylor 2003).

Hidden Harm (Gruer and Ainsworth 2003) cites the following potential impacts on children of problem drug use: emotional insecurity and impulsivity in young children; anti-social acts by boys; and depression, anxiety and withdrawal by girls. As children get older, conduct disorders, a risk of offending and alcohol or drug use become more likely; in teenagers, a risk of self-blame, guilt and increased suicide risk have all been reported.

Parents with moderate mental health problems are more likely than non-affected parents to perceive behavioural problems in their child, with about a half to two-thirds of children's behaviour being seen by them as affected (Tunnard 2004). However, this is based on parental perceptions, which are likely to be influenced by parental confidence as well as competence.

Some of the behaviours that might manifest in children who are affected by parental mental health problems or substance misuse can be seen as coping mechanisms. The research into coping strategies for children in these circumstances is limited and relates to more generic adverse circumstances, such as parental disability and domestic violence. Gorin (2004) identifies four ways of coping that emerge from the literature and research available (see box). These coping responses are more likely to emerge unconsciously than as deliberate strategies; and it is likely that ways of coping will change over time (Bancroft *et al.* 2004).

Coping mechanisms of children and young people whose parents have mental health/substance misuse/domestic violence problems

Avoidance/distraction

This can include physically avoiding parents or the home environment, with many children finding a 'haven', such as a friend or family members' home or their own bedroom (Mullender *et al.* 2002). Avoidance can also be psychological, with children ignoring or not thinking about their problems or pretending things are otherwise. Some children become loners or refuse to discuss their feelings. Others use distractions, such as music, TV, computers or (more often for girls than boys) writing in diaries (Fuller *et al.* 2000). Some children appear to throw themselves into their schoolwork or a hobby; some deflect attention from their real lives by making things up to tell their peers about their home life (Barnard and Barlow 2003). Ericksen and Henderson (1992) reported younger children talking to soft toys and pets and creating imaginary worlds.

Protection or inaction

Children can feel responsible for their parents' well-being or that of their siblings. One way this manifests itself in children is by them 'keeping watch' for signs of difficulty, which for some children can lead to staying away from school or avoiding going out. This is particularly noted in studies relating to parental mental health and to parental alcohol misuse. Girls are more commonly reported to take protective action in this way (Laybourn, Brown and Hill 1996). Where parental substance misuse is present, some children have spoken of hiding money or possessions and others of giving their parents money that they have saved for them. In all cases, when children don't take protective action they can experience feelings of guilt and distress about this, particularly (but not exclusively) when there is domestic violence or abuse of their siblings.

Confrontation/intervention/self-destruction

The most common way for children to intervene or confront their parents is by shouting at them (this is more likely than physical intervention in domestic violence situations). Some children dispense drugs, alcohol and/or medication to parents and others try psychological strategies to try and change their parent's behaviour or views, such as ridiculing them or appealing to them.

Help-seeking and action

Telling others about their situation or asking for advice from external sources is the second most common response by children (the most common being avoidance). Where children are able to discuss their situation this helps them to make sense of their own feelings and to be involved in considering the best way forward; both of which are factors known to increase their resilience. Unfortunately, when there is pressure to keep things secret within families, this undermines the potential for children to utilise this important coping behaviour.

Source: Gorin 2004

Identity

As children get older and become more curious about the world around them, developing clear likes, dislikes and opinions, there is a tendency for them to see themselves as being at the centre of everything. This is natural, but can be problematic when children have a disproportionate sense of their own impact and responsibility for what goes on around them. Where parental problems are seen as more clearly emanating from another source, for example when children view parental drinking as an 'illness', they are less likely to experience this sense of guilt and responsibility (Laybourn *et al.* 1996). However, broadly the research shows that parental substance misuse can erode self-esteem, self-worth and confidence (Taylor 2013). Additionally, a fear of developing the same problems as their parents is common in children affected by either parental substance use or parental mental health problems. For example many professionals encounter children who have discussed their fear that mental illness is 'catching'. Others may replicate their parent's behaviour as a way of connecting with their parent, 'thereby achieving some kind of closeness and identification' (Kroll and Taylor 2008 in Taylor 2013, p.10).

Children and young people who have a clear sense of themselves as separate from their families and their problems tend to fare better than children who don't. Developing a view of themselves as valued and special is an important part of this and can potentially be undermined by inconsistent parenting where there is a lack of positive reinforcement. At worst this can lead to children lacking confidence and feeling 'unlovable' (Fahlberg 1991).

Identity problems can be compounded further for black and minority ethnic children and children of dual heritage. Depending on their family's attitude and behaviour, children could potentially have a clear sense of their gender, race and culture by the age of three or four (Bee 2000), but this will vary. However, children may sometimes internalise racist stereotypes from the wider society and misattribute their parent's substance misuse to their ethnicity.

Where children and young people act as young carers of parents affected by substance misuse of mental health problems, it is important to acknowledge that there are some potentially beneficial aspects of the experience, with many feeling it to be a positive choice that bolsters their self-esteem and enhances their skills, maturity, relationships and emotional intelligence.

Family and social relationships

The impact on families of becoming isolated from extended families or wider networks of support has already been mentioned, but it is also possible for immediate family members to experience isolation from each other as a result of their difficulties. This can manifest itself in concrete ways, such as parental separation or divorce; or in more subtle ways, such as avoidance of each other or a lack of open communication.

There is often a tendency for parents to underplay their problems, either in an attempt to protect the child from knowing too much or as a result of denial. However, children often know more than their parents think they do and they pick up on things that, if denied, can lead to an increased sense of confusion and isolation. Such secrets and lies could be described as creating 'a world of mirrors where nothing is as it seems' (Kroll and Taylor 2003, p.184). If children (or partners) are not told the truth, and they suspect as much, they can experience this as rejection, become mistrustful and find their suspicions are raised further. They also may put their efforts into trying to investigate their suspicions (Houmoller et al. 2011). Denial within families can cause a range of reactions in children such as anger, blame and conflict or alliances and splits within the family.

Difficulties in communication can also take the form of inappropriate comments being made to children by parents when they are distressed, angry or inebriated.

Changes in family members' roles in response to changing situations over time (such as one parent taking over the role of the 'unwell' parent or children taking on 'adult' tasks) can lead to children and young people struggling with new ways of relating to family members. Later, when a parent is more able to take the reins again, this may be resisted and lead to conflict.

Children's friendships outside the family can suffer due to stigma, not feeling they can bring friends home and the responsibilities of their caring role. When faced with a crisis, some young people leave home prematurely, whereas others stay on longer than they might otherwise do, to support one or both parents or siblings. For young people who do wish to leave home, gaps in benefits can be prohibitive; similarly, for those who look after parents, a lack of financial resources and support can restrict access to some of the recreation and relaxation opportunities open to others.

Social presentation

The way in which children and young people present to others can be affected by parental difficulty. If there is poor hygiene or inappropriate dress due to neglect, children can appear different, experience bullying or show a lack of confidence. If parents model inappropriate behaviour or coping styles (such as aggression, substance use or criminal behaviour) and their children exhibit them, this will set them apart further resulting in people perceiving them negatively.

Self-care skills

Children and young people's self-care skills can similarly be reduced in these circumstances: a lack of guidance and support, or experiences of neglect, can result in a lack of self-esteem, low mood or lack of skills development. Conversely, the child undertaking caring responsibilities from a young age can heighten such skills.

To conclude, the literature on the potential impact on children of parental mental health and substance misuse continues to grow and is useful in highlighting the sorts of issues faced by children and their families. Assessing the impact on individual children and families is a skilled and complex task that relies on the analysis, reflection and self-awareness of those undertaking it to counter any assumptions or unchecked value judgements. A clear focus, which questions and explores the everyday experience of children and other family members in addition to a focus on crisis or 'unusual' incidents, is needed, along with a child-focused, ecological-transactional approach (which recognises the dynamic interplay between parental stress and child distress, which influence each other in turn) and knowledge of research and other evidence about effective or promising interventions. Approaches to assessment are considered further in Chapter 5.

3
What helps build resilience in these families?

Some children seem to be more affected by trauma in childhood than others. The term for the apparently increased ability to emerge from difficult situations without major negative impact on the individual is 'resilience'. This chapter considers factors that increase resilience and emphasises the importance of children being helped to sustain or develop a sense of self-efficacy and autonomy. It also considers familial and parenting characteristics that can enhance resilience. The chapter goes on to consider cultural connectedness, values and identity within the community, which can have positive effects on a child's resilience. It stresses that knowledge of resilience and all the points made above, when translated into practical support, can promote positive change.

Services have for a long time tended to focus on vulnerable children in terms of the 'risks of significant harm' that they face or the 'needs' they have that are not being met at the time. However, a focus on risks and needs alone does not make full use of our understanding of why some people overcome adversity and translating this into ways of supporting people (Galvani and Forrester 2009). This is recognised, and in recent years there has been a greater tendency (supported by the *Framework for the Assessment of Children in Need and their Families* (Department of Health 2000) and by the *Common Assessment Framework* (HM Government 2006)), to consider the strengths and protective factors within families. Indeed, the increased popularity of strengths-based approaches and models, for example, Signs of Safety,[1] are founded on this. This raises the question

---

1   The Signs of Safety is an innovative strengths-based, safety-organised approach to child protection casework. The model of its approach was created in Western Australia by Andrew Turnell and Steve Edwards. The approach has attracted international attention and is being used by many in North America, Europe and Australasia.

of what strengths or factors within individuals, families or the wider life experience of children enable some to cope better with adverse experiences, unmet needs or risks than others? Also, why do some children who experience abuse or neglect or parental alcohol misuse or who witness domestic violence appear to fare better than others who have had similar adverse experiences? What makes the difference? This apparently increased ability to emerge from difficult situations without major negative impacts on the individual is referred to as resilience.

The notion of 'resilience' within social care, particularly in relation to children's services, has gained increasing currency in recent years. Parrott *et al.* (2008) argue that the research around resilience has moved through different phases within that time, with more of a focus on individual factors initially, moving on to a focus on family factors and more recently taking a more ecological perspective, which considers the interactions between individuals and the social environment. The role of culture and the underpinning beliefs and values of individuals, families and communities can also influence the way in which people 'cope'.

Therefore, resilience factors operate at the level of the child, family, culture and external environment. There are different manifestations of 'resilience', for example there are those who succeed despite high-risk status, those who exhibit maturity and coping in the face of chronic stress and those who have suffered extreme trauma but have recovered and prospered (Newman and Blackburn 2002). Resilience is not fixed but changes over time, often showing itself in later life following an earlier phase where difficulties in coping were exhibited. That is because resilience is not a 'trait' but an interaction between an individual and their circumstances (Taylor 2013).

Whilst there is a lack of research into children's perspectives in relation to resilience (Templeton *et al.* 2006), the few longitudinal studies that have looked at outcomes over time show that many children recover from short-lived problems, but when adversities are continuous and severe and there are no observable protective factors, resilience is much rarer.

> …there is…no simple association between stress and gain. Some stressors may trigger resilient assets in children, others may compound chronic difficulties. If children are subjected to a relentless stream of multiple adversities, negative consequences are highly likely to follow. (Newman and Blackburn 2002, p.4)

Poor early experiences don't necessarily dictate future outcomes, however, as compensatory interventions can trigger responses that enhance resilience. For the purposes of this handbook the focus on resilience is synonymous with a focus on 'what's good for families' and especially 'what's good for the children within families'. It is concerned with what helps in minimising the impact of their difficulties and maximising the parent's opportunity to parent their child well enough and for the family to remain together. But this notion of resilience and a focus on it is not without its problems, and it is important to consider them here.

First, if measures of 'resilience' focus on tangible but arbitrary aspects of an individual's apparent progress in life – such as doing well academically or securing employment, having a busy social life or sustaining a long-term relationship – then they may miss the less visible factors that may be at play. For instance, the apparently 'high achiever' may be viewed as having survived their early experiences relatively unscathed, when in fact their emotional life, confidence or self-esteem may be affected in ways that are not seen, reported nor considered. The 'protective factors' or 'resilience' factors perceived by others to be present for the person may in fact mask harm or ways of 'coping' that may not be helpful in the long term (Galvani and Forrester 2009; Adamson and Templeton 2012). Equally, the lengths to which they have had to go in order to avoid some of the 'poorer outcomes' associated with adversity, may be great. It could be seen as minimising their struggle, or even offensive, to make statements that assume that in some way such individuals have been 'more resilient' or even 'coped better' than others.

Second, images that have been used to signify 'resilient children' as somehow 'unbreakable', 'bouncing back' or 'invulnerable' can be unhelpful (Rutter 1993, 1999) because resilience is relative, not absolute, and can change over time. Kroll and Taylor (2003) highlight the possibility of assumptions being made about a child that they are: 'once ok, always ok' (p.151). They discuss the potential for children who appear to be coping well at one time either to be concealing their difficulties or for their problems to be stored up for another time. At this point, they may become more vulnerable in a way that is compounded by their period of 'coping'. The positive labels of 'resilience' can therefore be as misleading as the negative ones.

Third, in contrast to the above, those who experience mental health problems – such as depression or post-traumatic stress as a result of their experiences – can be seen as having an appropriate response to their situation. Their emotional reaction is, perhaps, if viewed more positively, congruent, expressive and necessary. Such reactions may be a first step in helping some people to identify, question and move on from any damaging perceptions or self-beliefs that their experiences have left them with. Another example of this is when someone is perceived as 'immature', when in fact having the opportunity to be less mature than some of their peers (e.g. playing, having fun and spending time with friends) might be a necessary step for a child or young person who has experienced poor parenting or adversity (McCarthy and Galvani 2012).

Fourth, a focus on resilience could be interpreted as conferring too much responsibility on the person who has experienced the adversity, their 'hardiness' in relation to the adversity becoming the focus. This could in itself potentially compound any guilt, self-blame and sense of over-responsibility that individuals may experience.

Finally, Newman and Blackburn (2002) raise the issue of the tension that can occur between 'protection' and 'resilience' – to some extent, resilience can often be seen as occurring as a result of exposure to stress. They therefore suggest that an over-concentration on identifying and eliminating risk factors could potentially weaken children's capacity to overcome adversity. They would argue that gradual exposure to life's stresses at a manageable level (this would be hard to gauge) could help people/children develop a resistance to adverse reactions to stress. Parrott et al. (2008) also argue that resilience is present in all human beings and that its development involves learning and can be therapeutic, helping people develop emotional strength and capacity to cope with future life events. Nonetheless, experiences that could be seen to promote resilience would not always be socially acceptable. In relation to child protection issues, if children were left to cope with some situations in order to 'build their resistance to adversity', this would be extremely contentious, potentially very dangerous and clearly unethical. But it is important to acknowledge that all interventions, even when (or perhaps especially when) their purpose is to protect, can either harm or help. A useful perspective to help with such dilemmas can be to remind ourselves that the purpose of services and interventions should be to elicit the internal strengths, resilience, motivations and goals that already exist within individuals, families and communities.

Also, given some of the other concerns about the notion of resilience, it is important to be clear in our thinking and in what we communicate when we talk about resilience with other professionals, in reports and with families. It is not so much about someone's capacity to manage as it is about the associations between the presence of some factors (often referred to as 'protective factors') with long-term, good outcomes.

To assess resilience factors alongside risks, and to give full consideration to factors and interventions likely to promote resilience and reduce risks, increases the opportunity for establishing a way forward that is, comprehensive, evidence-informed and promotes 'best-possible' outcomes. Such a focus can help reduce the sorts of 'additional harm' that can compound difficult experiences, perhaps needlessly, when some attention given to an aspect of someone's life or needs could relieve their situation or distress. The risk/vulnerability matrix on page 87 provides a useful framework for this.

Much work has been done to explore what factors seem to support the resilience of individuals and these factors will be described in the following sections. However, it is not enough to identify what factors are associated with resilience. This information only becomes useful if such factors can be affected, and such knowledge can be translated into effective service responses, support or interventions for children, families and communities.

Factors that increase resilience

The parenting, familial and community factors that seem to improve outcomes, if present for children and young people, are considered separately in this section. In reality these factors often overlap.

Much of the literature and research about resilience or 'protective factors' (defined by Adamson and Templeton (2012, p.53) as 'a factor or process [which] reduces or prevents the impact of [a] risk factor') refers to adversity in a general sense, though it is still relevant for children affected specifically by parental mental health or parental substance misuse. Newman and Blackburn (2002), in their international study, found that common factors could be seen across cultural and geographical boundaries. Other research has been more specific, such as Velleman's (1993, 2004) work on outcomes for children of alcohol-misusing parents or Parrott *et al.* (2008) and Taylor's (2013) overviews of the research relating to parental mental health and parental substance misuse respectively and Adamson and Templeton's (2012) work relating to children exposed to parental alcohol misuse. These, along with a range of sources, have been drawn on to compile the lists of resilience-enhancing factors below, including Velleman and Orford (1993, 1999), Newman and Blackburn (2002), McCarthy and Galvani (2012), Tunnard (2002a), Bancroft et al. (2004), Kroll and Taylor (2003) and Cleaver et al. (1999, 2011).

Factors that enhance children's resilience
Positive relationship with a family member or parental figure

For all children and young people facing difficulties of any kind, supportive family members are the most powerful positive factor influencing their ability to cope. This is due both to the attachment relationship, which provides the child with the foundation for their self-esteem and for developing relationships with others, and the increased likelihood of them receiving the care and support they need practically and emotionally.

The presence of at least one unconditionally supportive parent or parent substitute is key. Those who have a strong attachment relationship with their mothers are more likely to seek social support as a coping strategy (Taylor 2013). Similarly, young children who spend a lot of time with their fathers tend to have better outcomes in relation to school, friendships, self-esteem and life satisfaction (Lam et al. 2012 in Fatherhood Institute 2013). A strong attachment relationship enables children and young people to develop what Fonagy et al. (1994) refer to as a 'reflective self-function' (which they define as having an awareness of mental processes in oneself and in others, and the ability to take account of one's own mental states and those of others to understand why people behave in certain ways – in other words thinking about yourself in relation to others). Whilst the parent or parents who are experiencing substance misuse or mental health problems may provide the child with much of this understanding, the research indicates that the presence of another adult improves outcomes. Such adults do not necessarily have to live with the child, but need to be an integral and influential part of their lives. Often the partner of the parent who has the most difficulties is concerned about, or supporting, their partner. Their attention can be drawn away from the child, so this lends weight to the crucial need to support the 'least vulnerable' parent to bolster their ability to provide essential attention to the child. As Forrester and Harwin (2006 in Taylor 2013) point out, in the case of parental substance misuse, the non-using parent/partner may only act as a protective factor insofar as they are able to provide a warm response to the child, despite the stresses they are under (Forrester and Harwin 2006 in Taylor 2013).

Influence of another stable adult figure or figures

Beyond the child's family or home environment, the presence of a committed mentor or positive and interested adult outside the family is also an important positive factor. Such a relationship can provide the child or young person with encouragement, much-needed attention, consistency, a sense of stability and more. This may come from either informal networks such as members of the wider family, neighbours or friends' parents or from more formal sources such as teachers or other professionals. Such people can be an important source of support to parents by either giving them a break through the relief of knowing someone else is helping the child or providing a stabilising influence on the parent.

Positive social support networks and a social role

Support networks such as friendships, clubs and membership of groups or attendance at faith-based institutions can all help children develop a sense of being valued or 'valuable'. Participation in extracurricular activities, which children enjoy or are good at, can promote their self-esteem. Similarly, the opportunity for older children (through voluntary or part-time work or membership of supportive groups or organisations) to 'make a difference' by helping others enhances their self-esteem, social skills and the development of a positive identity.

Positive experiences away from the home can counter some of the stress or difficulty that some children face, giving them 'compensatory' moments of pleasure, fun and relaxation and something to look forward to. Having the opportunity to find out about how other people respond to them and to explore interests and skills in such settings, are all important in forming a sense of identity.

Positive, nurturing school experiences

This is linked with the above two points in terms of the opportunity schools provide for forming friendships with peers and other adults and for developing social skills, interests, talents and self-esteem. Educational success is an additional factor, which if experienced is associated with children who fare better later in life due to the opportunities it gives them, as well as to the increased self-esteem, knowledge and ways of understanding the world that help them to interact more positively within it.

A sense that one's own efforts can make a difference

For children as well as adults, their problems are likely to have a more negative impact on them if they feel helpless and that nothing is within their control. If they can be enabled to exert any influence on their own circumstances, however small, this can enhance their well-being. Being helped to make choices, and being consulted and asked about what they think will help them or what is important to them, can all promote their sense that they can make a difference. This links in with another important factor: the capacity to recognise and acknowledge the beneficial effects of adversity (as well as the damaging aspects). This may seem strange, but most people can relate to a sense that people often have when they have been through difficult times, that something within them has 'grown' or developed as a result. Whilst negative experiences aren't to be minimised, the impact of all experiences is mixed, and to acknowledge the positive can be affirming and help growth. Also, a sense that problems can be overcome is very important to young people becoming proactive and optimistic in their approach to life.

Personal or 'inherent' qualities

Children with good verbal skills, good cognitive ability, the absence of neurobiological problems and who demonstrate autonomy, sociability and good self-esteem tend to fare better than children who do not have these qualities. The extent to which some of these 'qualities' can be influenced varies, of course, and the absence of some of the factors may be compounded or caused by the problems children have faced in their lives. A child's behaviour, confidence and ability are not static, however. With support and opportunities, some children who are regarded as 'unsociable' or 'inarticulate' for example, may demonstrate significant changes over time.

A child's own 'coping' skills

The more children are able to understand and express their feelings, the more they can make sense of their situations and survive them with less harm done. In families where feelings are denied, where emotions are seen as volatile or silenced, it is much harder for children to develop such positive responses. Interventions that bolster a child's ability to recognise and name feelings, as well as to express them and ask for help, will enhance their resilience. Some social situations and opportunities, such as activities that are challenging but achievable, can also provide children with opportunities to develop coping skills.

A child's view of themselves and their circumstances

Children who see themselves as separate from the problems in their family tend to fare better than those who believe that they are a part of the problems and that their problems are a part of them. Children whose parents are distressed, unwell or intoxicated or in withdrawal, often, and understandably, think that they are somehow compounding or causing the problems that they see around them. Some children at times blame themselves for their parents' state or internalise their parents' feelings as being somehow about something they are or are not doing. Also, children feel the stigma that such families experience. They can feel alienated and judged and go on to internalise these negative views. Children who, while knowing they are part of a family, see themselves as distinct individuals with separate feelings, qualities and potential are likely to have better outcomes. Furthermore, where children have some insight and understanding into the difficulties their parent faces and are able to recognise when their parents are making positive changes, this can also be helpful to them (McCarthy and Galvani 2012).

Plans for the future

Children who can imagine their futures and who are encouraged and supported to make positive plans about their future are more likely to do well. Plans in the short term are also important, as they provide things to look forward to, both with and without the rest of their family.

Early and compensatory experiences

Where a parent has discrete episodes of mental illness with fairly high functioning in between episodes, this appears to increase the opportunity for resilience in the child, whereas those whose parents' problems are chronic and enduring are more negatively affected. Also, the older the child is at the onset of their parent's mental health problems, the greater the range of coping resources they will have developed by the time the problems start. Therefore less early exposure to problems increases their life chances.

Similarly for children of substance-misusing parents, the absence of early loss and trauma will have given them the opportunity to develop their coping resources. Where there are substantial periods in which parents care for them well and they feel loved, they will fare better than if neglect is chronic and long term. Conversely, where levels of care and support differ significantly over time, with such changes making no sense to the child and messages about the value of the child being confusing, this will be more detrimental to children.

Familial and parenting characteristics that enhance resilience

A confiding relationship with a partner or with others

When parents under stress have a partner with whom they can share their thoughts, feelings and experiences and can be honest, their well-being and in turn their parenting capacity is enhanced. For lone parents or parents in less positive relationships, it is important to find a confidante elsewhere. Also, parents who have positive relationships with others are more likely to be able to develop a positive attachment with their child. Being able to listen to their partners or others and reciprocate within relationships enhances this further.

Cohesive parental relationship

The absence of parental conflict is associated with better outcomes for children. If parents are able to present a 'united front' to their children, showing that they agree and are consistent in the boundaries they set and the plans they have, this helps children by providing the consistency they need and reducing confusion, insecurity and uncertainty. Consistently enforced rules are another resilience factor within parenting; and a cohesive relationship (where there is more than one parent) will support this.

Parental self-esteem

Parents who (with or without support) are able to value themselves and see what their positive qualities and abilities are and what they mean to other people are better able to parent effectively. Therefore interventions and informal support that seek to enhance (rather than undermine) self-esteem are very important. Self-help groups have been found to help 'foster self determination' and promote self-esteem in adults with mental health problems (Burti et al. 2005 in Parrot et al. 2008). Additionally, adults who are 'optimistic' – expecting that things will probably turn out OK – seem to be more able to 'engage with protective processes', in turn promoting resilience (Parrott *et al.* 2008, p.6).

Social life, rituals and routines

Parents who have regular contact with other adults or families whom they value and enjoy being with are associated with greater resilience. Such opportunities, all too often lacking for families under stress, can enhance self-esteem and reduce stress. Obviously, if socialising tends to reinforce problematic drinking or substance use, or is with people or in settings that increase anxiety, this becomes detrimental, but enhancing the positive social opportunities available is important.

If families can manage to do some things together – such as going to the park or sitting down for a family meal – these positive and reliable experiences can enhance relationships and children's self-esteem and outlook, and give positive memories. Observing special occasions and rituals that were previously adhered to, such as all gathering together while a child opens their birthday presents, is important even when (and especially because) life is chaotic and littered with crises, as are the maintenance of consistent family rules.

Adequate finances and employment opportunities

Families who have sufficient finances available to them fare better than those who don't. Increased resources mean more access to support for individuals within the family or for the whole family. These resources include: more suitable housing; social and leisure opportunities; breaks and respite; private counselling; and access to support with childcare or even with domestic tasks. Where there is parental substance misuse, some of the areas of potential concern, such as finances being directed into drugs rather than in meeting children's basic needs, are mitigated if resources are more plentiful. However, this may mean in some families that it is easier to hide substance use, meaning some of the more emotional impacts on children, for example secrecy and denial, are harder to pick up.

Employment can obviously be one way of enhancing the finances of some families, and part-time work for women with mental health problems is known to be a protective factor (and, of course to reduce social isolation), but, conversely, full-time work for women with young children increases the risks of parental stress impacting negatively on children.

Constructive coping styles and deliberate parental actions to minimise adversity for children

The coping strategies employed by parents impact directly or indirectly on the way the child manages their experiences and emotions. Tunnard (2002a) reported on a Scottish study that demonstrated this link in families where parents were depressed. For example, if the parent had a non-productive coping style or avoided their problems (worrying, not talking about problems, self-blaming or wishful thinking) and was therefore less likely to seek help, their children tended to do the same. Conversely, if parents were more productive (focusing on positives, dealing with problems, seeking help), children did the same.

Some parents are proactive in trying to minimise the impact of their problems on their children. Parents who have experienced mental health problems over time and have come to know what helps and hinders their well-being often develop strategies to minimise the stress on them and to get support when they need it. Tunnard (2002a) reported on some of the strategies adopted by substance-misusing parents, which included planned separations as a way of protecting the child from their drug use or inability to care sufficiently well for them at the time. Often this meant the child spending time with relatives (frequently maternal grandmothers) for a period instead. Other strategies included safe storage of equipment; keeping other drug users out of the home or having rules about not using drugs when the children were around. These strategies worked better for some people than others. Other strategies adopted by parents to reduce their own health problems arising from their drug use and, in turn, reduce the negative impact on their parenting included not taking drugs daily, getting enough sleep, eating properly, taking iron tablets and trying to avoid stress.

Parental substance misuse in itself can be viewed as a coping strategy when it has developed as a way of numbing feelings or avoiding problems. It is important that if people are being encouraged to reduce or abstain from substance or alcohol use, alternative coping strategies are explored.

Receiving treatment

The effective management of any parental mental health problems is an important protective factor. In relation to parental substance misuse, an acknowledgement of the problem and its effects in the home is also a positive factor (Taylor 2013). Additionally, there is some evidence that going into treatment for substance problems and using a substitute such as methadone can be a significant protective factor, leading to far greater stability, predictability of daily life and reduction of the distractions, secrecy and denial that impact on parenting and on children. Some parents, however, fear that if they use substitutes they will develop another addiction (Tunnard 2002a). It is also interesting to note that parents whose children live with them tend to do well in treatment (NTA 2012), which could be because of the added motivation they feel to recover from their problems for their children. This illustrates the transactional nature of not only needs and risks but also of protective factors between parents and their children.

Receiving treatment or therapy for any psychological difficulty can mean raising memories and feelings that have been buried or denied as a coping mechanism, so undergoing treatment for complex problems linked with substance misuse or mental health problems can have an impact that is potentially negative in the shorter term. Ultimately, however, if such interventions are made in a timely fashion, and if they are followed through by the individual concerned, they should promote resilience.

Openness and good communication

Whatever the nature of the problems within families, if there is an atmosphere of openness in which thoughts, feelings and uncertainties can be safely expressed, the outcomes for children (and the wider family) will be supported by this. In their review of resilience factors in relation to children of alcohol-misusing families, McCarthy and Galvani (2012) make the point that it is 'vital' that there is open communication about parents' alcohol use instead of 'tip-toeing' around the subject (p.8).

A knowledge of 'protective factors'

It is logical and has been demonstrated (Velleman 2004) that if parents know about the things that make a difference to children and to the outcomes for them, they are more able to utilise them. Helping parents to recognise the importance of certain factors, such as children's engagement in hobbies or the importance of observing family occasions, keeping some routines and consistent family rules, is helpful and potentially empowering.

Community factors that enhance resilience

Cultural connectedness, values and identity

Families who see themselves as part of their community and who are linked in with groups and services fare better than those who are disconnected, as already discussed in Chapter 2. For example if a positive identity or valued local culture exists within a community, or a family identifies positively as members of an ethnic or religious group, this relates to better outcomes and a more positive individual and family identity.

A socially rich environment in which people are inclined to look out for each other, intervene and help out is associated with better outcomes for children and families, as are good community resources such as accessible childcare, healthcare, transport, leisure and education facilities.

Bolstering resilience

As stated earlier, knowledge of resilience or 'protective' factors is not in itself enough to influence the experiences of children. However, if such knowledge is translated into support and actions aimed directly at influencing such factors, this can promote positive change. At the individual level, this could mean placing more emphasis on facilitating a child's access to a supportive adult or social or leisure opportunity or helping a parent understand and act on the knowledge of what is important for their child. When it comes to planning and shaping services, such knowledge adds weight to the importance of supporting extended family members, working more proactively with fathers and linking responses more effectively with schools or community resources. As, on the whole, the literature shows informal support to be more helpful to families than formal professional involvement, it is also worth services considering how they can better:

...foster the characteristics of responsiveness, flexibility, reliability and supportiveness that characterise family and community supports. (Olsen and Wates 2003, p.26)

Some resilience factors are more amenable to influence than others and it would be naïve to suggest that a focus on boosting resilience factors alone will fully address the problems that many families face. However, an awareness of resilience factors and a weighing up of these alongside a consideration of needs, risks and potential for change will enhance assessments and could give rise to more appropriate interventions.

In conclusion, this focus on resilience can provide a helpful framework for guiding direct work with children and families experiencing complex challenges such as parental substance misuse or/and parental mental health problems. Examining factors that can act separately and together to boost resilience can help practitioners to identify possible routes and ideas for engaging with and supporting children and families to address their needs.

4
Professional responses and barriers to effective practice

This chapter explores the barriers, at the practice and strategic levels, to effective responses by services. It considers the practice level, where too few professionals think about the family, the impacts of one member on another and opportunities to promote and use the support of friends and family members. It looks at the lack of interagency knowledge sharing and the uncertainty amongst professionals as to how and where to access specific knowledge and expertise. It suggests that a greater focus on critical reflection and support with analysis is needed. It goes on to consider why some service responses are proving unhelpful, including the lack of focus on fathers, and some of the reasons why families may be reluctant to use a service.

This chapter also considers the strategic level and why services are often organised around discrete areas – such as 'mental health' or 'substance misuse' – despite these not being separate and distinct for individuals and families. It suggests that more integrated working needs to be instigated, while keeping to tight budgets and appropriate levels of access to services.

Barriers to effective practice: What gets in the way?

This chapter explores, in more depth, some of the key practice and strategic issues of relevance to those providing support and services on an individual or family level.

Chapter 1 discussed the general tendency towards too little or late intervention sometimes leading to more extreme responses further down the line. Whilst some of these issues, such as the lack of talking therapies available for those with mild or moderate mental health difficulties, can be seen as linked to a lack of resources, others are directly affected by deficits in practitioner awareness, knowledge, training and confidence. These issues, preceded by a focus on the issue of stigma, are discussed in Part 1 of this chapter.

Chapter 1 also established that the way in which services currently respond to families affected by parental mental health problems and substance misuse is variable and that there is a lack of preventative and early intervention services (despite policy drivers aimed at promoting them). There are also significant barriers to providing coordinated support across relevant professional disciplines, with interagency working difficulties being rife and perhaps the hardest factor to overcome. Part 2 of this chapter focuses on such issues, which are most appropriately and meaningfully addressed at a strategic level.

Raising awareness and challenging stigma
The nature and impact of stigma

> Having a mental illness is one of the most overtly stigmatised attributes an individual can have, rivalled only by substance abuse or homelessness. (Link *et al.* 1999 in Hinshaw 2005, p.716)

The stigmatisation of people with mental health problems and substance misuse issues is well documented, and its significance and impact on families has been discussed to some extent earlier in this book. Stigmatisation does not occur as a result of the presence of mental illness or substance misuse, but as a result of the discriminatory attitudes and responses of wider society to them.

Experiences of stigmatisation compound people's difficulties significantly and can limit opportunities, such as their access to housing, employment, medical care and insurance coverage (Corrigan 2004), and is the greatest barrier to social inclusion for people with mental health problems (Social Exclusion Unit 2004). Stigma can also limit the availability of research funding, access to treatment and attainment of personal relationships and educational and vocational goals (Sartorius 1998).

Both substance misuse and mental health problems are not necessarily visible, so stigma and (perceived or anticipated) negative attitudes can lead people to conceal their diagnosis or difficulties and make them less likely to ask for help or admit to the nature of their problems. The negative media portrayal of those who misuse substances and those with mental health problems as dangerous or potentially violent (Wahl 1995) further influences public perception and, in turn, the view that those with mental health or substance use problems have about others and about themselves. As Hinshaw puts it, prejudice, stereotyping and discrimination are related, but stigma:

> …incorporates all these processes but transcends them by including the strong likelihood that the castigated individual will internalise the degradation. (Hinshaw 2005, p.715)

Unfortunately, most of the relevant literature and research relating to people with mental health or substance misuse issues focuses on the negative rather than any positive aspects of people or their lives.

> …whilst nearly all of the relevant literature has emphasised family burden – relating to the negative effects of coping with a relative with mental illness – anecdotal evidence suggests that in a subset of families, the experience has fostered sensitivity, courage, and a more positive outlook on life. (Hinshaw 2005, p.721)

Part 1: The practice level
Awareness/knowledge and confidence

The reasons for a lack of awareness (of issues that if better understood would enhance practice responses) are complex, but in part, the separation of services means too few relevant practitioners and professionals think in terms of family relationships and the impacts of one member on another. The pattern of client contact within adult drug services and in some adult mental health settings, for example, makes it easy to lose sight of the needs (or even the presence or relevance) of the adult's child or children. Some agencies discourage adult users from bringing children into the office (or service setting) because facilities aren't 'suitable' or because of understandable concerns that the child's presence will impinge on what can be discussed. However, in making such decisions or responses, agencies should consider far more than simple issues of 'practicality', since this approach may critically skew what is looked at (in terms of needs of the family) and significantly narrow the focus of what is seen or noticed by the professional.

Kroll and Taylor (2003) interviewed practitioners from a range of the relevant settings and found that many of those working with adults felt that parenting capacity was not something they could assess. Furthermore, there was often ambivalence or uncertainty among them (and it seems likely to be the case for many non-statutory children's services as well) about making referrals to statutory children and families social work teams for them to assess parenting capacity and needs. Many were unsure about when or how to make a referral and, in particular, whether or not they were able to make an informal enquiry without 'triggering the might of the child protection machinery' (p.225). Furthermore, Ofsted (2011), in their analysis of case reviews, found that drug and alcohol services 'often overlooked the parenting capacity of their clients or didn't recognise the important contribution their service could make to decision-making about their client's child' (p.21).

Conversely, many children's services practitioners consider parental mental health problems or substance misuse to be specialist areas falling outside their expertise. Neither do they appear, however, to be involving (or to be successful in attempts to involve) relevant adult workers within their processes as often as they could. Forrester and Harwin (2006) found substance use workers to be conspicuously absent from interagency meetings, for example.

The extent to which working in this way, solely with individuals, has become fixed in many services should not be underestimated. For many practitioners and professionals used to working in centres with adults only, visiting people at home or working across family boundaries can be perceived, for example, as unethical or potentially damaging to professional/adult service user relationships or confidentiality.

That said, increased knowledge and confidence can only be advantageous for practice. Whilst no one professional discipline can hold expertise or knowledge in all relevant issues, better awareness of where and with whom expertise or knowledge is held and how to access it is essential.

So it seems that, before the knowledge gaps of relevant professionals can be addressed, there is a need for increased awareness and appreciation of the systemic nature of family functioning – the impact that one family member and their needs and behaviour has on another – as well as a clearer message within organisations that supporting families is everybody's responsibility.

Mental health awareness

Tunnard (2004) highlighted the need for a greater understanding of mental health issues and for all professionals to understand that the vast majority of people with mental health problems don't harm or neglect their children, and that fluctuations in their parenting capacity could in many cases be accommodated by flexible services. Also, practitioners and professionals need to value and recognise the importance of wider family and friends more, and to utilise and promote such sources of support more routinely in their work with families.

Drug and alcohol awareness

Velleman (2004), in his work concerning substance misuse, discussed the need for those working with children in all settings to be made aware of the possible signs and symptoms that can manifest themselves in children who are adversely affected by parental substance use or other parental problems – such as behavioural and emotional difficulties, school problems, difficulty with transitions to adolescence. He also argued the need for a greater awareness of resilience factors among professionals and parents.

The nature of substance misuse and responses to it are developing all the time, so there is a particular challenge in raising the awareness and confidence of relevant professionals in this area. Forrester and Harwin (2006) identified a need for more training around substance misuse for social workers in child care. Lack of confidence was raised, by Kroll and Taylor (2003), as potentially contributing to the reasons for a lack of joint intervention, along with professional 'fears of exposing one's practice' to professionals from other disciplines (p.271).

In their work with two local authorities, Hart and Powell (2006) also identified that both social workers and referrers appeared to lack an understanding of the complexity of assessing the impact of, and the needs arising from, parental drug misuse. A number of referrals, case notes and reports said no more than 'drug use by parents', and gave no adequate consideration or information to consider critically the variables of the individual family situation. This was often done without consulting drug workers, who may have had expertise to offer. They also found that many workers had naïve views about drugs and tended to overemphasise abstinence as being required rather than having a clear and critical focus on children's needs. Elliot and Watson (1998) highlighted that many parents think workers don't know enough about their difficulties or about polydrug use and focus too narrowly on heroin use.

Assessment issues

There is often a lack of clear analytical assessment of families' needs, with a tendency (found by Hart and Powell (2006) prior to the introduction of the 'single assessment') for repeated initial assessments to take place following single incidents of concern and often no core assessments taking place until increased professional intervention was necessitated through the family situation worsening. When assessments do take place, they tend to be undertaken on a single-agency basis with inadequate consultation with other relevant professionals. Plans for interventions often fail to utilise the network of potential support and input. Hart and Powell (2006) found partnership working to be underdeveloped, with little use being made of network meetings or family group conferences.

Social work assessments that take place within the *Framework for the Assessment of Children in Need and their Families* (Department of Health 2000) have often been found: to lack narrative; to be parent-focused, with children being less visible than they ought to be; and to lack transparent and clear analysis (Dalzell and Sawyer 2007; Hart and Powell 2006). This is not just true of assessments relating to families affected by parental mental health issues or substance misuse but of all family assessments: the struggle to establish what is 'good enough' in terms of parenting, when significant harm is indicated, and how to achieve good outcomes within resource constraints applies to them all. Yet poor assessments take almost as much, if not the same amount, of time and energy as good ones. A greater focus on critical reflection and support with analysis is needed and, ultimately, may well reduce the efforts required by professionals.

Decision-making

Decision-making often happens almost by default. Kroll and Taylor (2003) found that factors that influenced assessments and decisions – not necessarily consciously at the time – include the reputation of the family, a fear of making judgements when there is poverty and anxiety about the impact of child protection work. They also found a tendency for professionals to feel relieved when some families withdrew from services and to be more disposed to close such cases or withdraw the service in response to apparent withdrawal. The lack of clear analysis and critical consideration of family circumstances over time can, and often does, lead to decisions and interventions that occur almost 'by accident'. Such cases include children becoming 'looked after' in crisis but at a time when the situation is no longer amenable to change, so they end up remaining away from home after months of uncertainty. When kinship carers look after the child, this lack of clear planning, direction and support can place greater strain on the placement too. Hollows (2003) used the term 'creeping judgements (p.69)' to describe these kinds of situation – where, for example, a series of short-term, 'duty' responses set the pattern and nature of long-term intervention, even though they are often based on single incidents or 'snapshot' assessments. In similar vein, the DfE-commissioned review of social workers' decision-making at the front door argues that: 'the complexity of social workers' decision-making is increased by the fact that many sequential decisions have to be made throughout the day, which engenders depletion or decision fatigue' (Kirkman and Melrose 2014, p.4).

Unhelpful service responses

Assessing what support is needed by families and finding the resources or skills to provide whatever is necessary are not easy tasks. However, some approaches seem particularly unhelpful, such as the use of 'warning letters' in which it is 'threatened' that assessments will take place if further incidents are heard of or referrals received, or offering early morning appointments and then closing the case if a family doesn't attend. Such practices are seen as an intervention and yet they don't facilitate an assessment taking place and potentially hinder current or future engagement with some families. It is not surprising that many professionals, not used to taking a whole-family approach, perhaps do not know how to intervene for the best and are more likely to rely on more mechanised uncritical responses, which seem 'safer', regardless of their effectiveness. Jack (1997) asks where in the 'present blaming culture' for social work 'is the incentive and support for social workers to take risks in developing less intrusive and more supportive approaches to work with families' (p.116).

Much is often made by professionals of parents 'refusing services' or 'failing to admit their problems'. Hamer (2005) argues that such statements are labelling and are often based on professionals' notions of 'support', when what families are actually refusing are interventions that don't meet their needs. These may, in the view of parents, have intended or unintended consequences, which place greater strain on their families or which they don't understand because they have not been generated through any meaningful collaboration with them. Services are often offered by professionals who are suggesting to parents that they are not managing or that things need to change or improve. This can make it very hard for some parents to accept what is being offered, as it may be construed as an admission of 'not coping', which brings a whole range of anxieties, many of which are valid, with it. As Bostock *et al.* (2005) point out, all too often in social care organisations, 'learning' is based around blame and condemnation of individuals. Therefore it is not surprising that individual workers are constantly aware of and averse to risk.

Parental 'resistance' to intervention and support is not necessarily caused by professional ways of working and is common among people experiencing addictions. However, apart from substance misuse workers, most professionals get little or no preparation within their training for working with denial, minimisation, avoidance or aggression and this makes them less likely to respond in ways that reduce resistance. In fact, much of the way in which child protection work is conducted would seem likely to increase resistance.

Lack of focus on fathers

A tendency within social care and family support services to focus interventions on mothers and to exclude fathers can reduce the usefulness of practice and services (NSPCC Information Service 2015). In assessments of need as well as within interventions, the focus, even when initially targeted at the whole family, quickly shifts to a focus on the mother (Ryan 2000). This was borne out in case file audits (Roskill *et al.* 2008 in Fatherhood Institute 2013), which found less than half of involved birth fathers were invited to meetings that took place as part of the assessment process. This means that not only do fathers miss out on the opportunity to better understand and meet their children's needs, but also mothers are ascribed the lion's share of responsibility for changing family circumstances. Another potential impact of this is to fail to provide support for (or even to collude with) situations where mothers or children are afraid of fathers, for example where there is domestic violence. As Kroll and Taylor (2003) point out, if professionals are reticent about approaching fathers, this must disempower mothers further. This failure to include fathers as a matter of course further undermines a whole-family approach that could improve the effectiveness of interventions.

There are a number of ways in which failures to involve fathers effectively in assessments and interventions undermine the success of the work and fail to address risks to children. An NSPCC review, *Hidden Men* (NSPCC Information Service 2015), of serious case reviews since 2008 indicated failures to identify and work with men to have been a significant factor in what went wrong. The case reviews took place as a result of either physical or sexual abuse by a male carer/father or the murder of a child by a father with mental health problems. A range of factors were seen to be at play and contributing to these failures.

- Professionals working with fathers/male carers (e.g. mental health or substance misuse services) did not communicate about potential risks in relation to these men with professionals working with the child. In some cases this may have been because they were unaware of the man's contact with the child/children.

- An overreliance on mothers to report on circumstances relating to the father/male rather than checking this out and exploring things more widely with extended family and others.

- Professionals not wanting to pry or be seen as 'judgemental' can be reluctant to ask too many questions of or relating to men who get into what may be perceived as short-term relationships with mothers.

- The ability of estranged fathers/significant men to provide safe care, stability and protection to children whose mothers may be struggling to do so can be overlooked or ignored. Additionally, men may have key information and knowledge to share that is not elicited, which significantly undermines the quality of assessment and subsequent responses.

There may be a number of reasons for the above failures. Some explain it in terms of men's reluctance to engage, often being 'wary of authority', lacking confidence in talking with female professionals or feeling that 'family work is women's business' (Fatherhood Institute 2013, p.3). However, Roskill *et al.*'s (2008) research showed that when men were invited to attend meetings 75 per cent did so. The Fatherhood Institute (2013) argue that professionals within children and families services can tend to operate from a 'deficit' perspective in relation to men and fathers, 'dismissing, ignoring or failing to reach out to them' (p.4). They argue that this perspective is underpinned by beliefs (identified by Hawkins and Dollahite in 1997) that men don't love their children as much as mothers do, are unwilling or unable to change and are less relevant than mothers to a child's development. Additionally, they suggest there is an underpinning belief that men/fathers generally pose a risk. The Fatherhood Institute point out, critically, that operating from a deficit perspective can result in professionals 'overvaluing' positive behaviour in fathers and thereby underestimating risk (Brandon *et al.* 2011 in Fatherhood Institute 2013).

Further to the above, Darryl Dugdale (cited in *Community Care*, May 2012) found in his work on this issue that practitioners' responses to 'masculinity' often go unchecked, with the tendency for some to see men generally as 'unpredictable or violent'. He argues that more attention should be paid to how men explain their behaviour and 'unpick' situations and how they understand any harm they may be causing. The likelihood is that there are numerous factors at play. However, it is clear that whatever the cause of failures to engage with men, the result is the reduced effectiveness of work aimed at enhancing the welfare of children and protecting them.

> Serious case reviews repeatedly found that although men around a child who died had posed a risk, this had not been identified or acted upon, and that men who could have been a resource often had information that agencies would have found helpful in understanding the child's situation if only they had been in touch or had been listened to (Ofsted 2011; Brandon *et al.* 2011). (Fatherhood Institute 2013, p.4)

Practical arrangements

The practical arrangements within which many services operate can also be seen as hindering effective practice, for example a lack of flexibility about where and when appointments can take place. This can mean that some parents who are already known to be struggling with structure or appointments are potentially being 'set up to fail' if they are only offered early morning appointments or given lots of appointments at different places (and especially if these are without adequate facilities for their children). In some cases, this is perhaps deliberate – some 'testing out' often occurs within the social work relationship and can provide useful information – but with some parents it could also reduce the possibility of securing a trusting, constructive relationship and of moving forward. Waiting times for appointments and assessments, a lack of mutual trust and a fear of children being removed are all further barriers to the take-up of services by parents.

Part 2: The strategic level
Complex range of 'single-user' services

Where there are parental mental health problems, the affected parent might be eligible for an assessment and services from an adult mental health team. Their child, if they have their own needs or difficulties, may have their needs assessed by a children and families social work team or a child and adolescent mental health service (CAMHS). Similarly, there are separate teams and services set up to assess and provide services for adults with substance misuse issues. Sometimes these are also aimed at those with problem alcohol use and at other times these are separate. Add in providers of education, community care services, health, therapeutic support, housing, probation and targeted youth support services and any one family could have a large number of agencies involved at one time. There are exceptions, as some services such as Troubled Families teams are set up with the whole family in mind, but even these services are usually one of a number of agencies involved in a family's life. Conversely, with no single route for support and differing realms of 'responsibility' within services, some individuals and families do not receive the support they require, with different services each thinking they are the responsibility of another.

Whilst services are often organised around discrete areas of need, such as 'mental health' or 'substance use', the needs of individuals and families are not separate and distinct. They often come with multiple problems such as poverty, child behavioural issues or domestic violence, and one area of difficulty compounds another, making such distinctions potentially misleading. In cases where there is dual diagnosis, the barriers to a seamless, integrated service are even greater. All too frequently, in the absence of clear guidance and proactive planning for responding to people with overlapping needs such as substance misuse and mental health problems, there is a tension between services that are primarily set up to deal with one issue or 'service user type'. For example, where mental ill health and substance misuse occur together, practitioners have told us of the pressure they encounter to 'narrow their vision' to the focus that is considered to be within their agency remit and therefore 'separate issues falsely'. Similarly, in certain circumstances, in order to ensure service users are viewed as meeting threshold criteria, there can be an increased emphasis on trying to find information to support the fact that a service user 'fits a label' so they can access the service.

Practitioners have talked to us about the disputes that often take place between services as to where the responsibility for the service user lies and how the work should proceed. For example, some hold the view that a person's substance use needs to be addressed before their mental health problems can be treated effectively, but for others, it's vice versa. It is more useful to work towards a model where mental health services are able to access or include support for those with drug or alcohol misuse problems and vice versa. There are also differences in opinion within different services regarding confidentiality and where the boundaries lie. In short, dual diagnosis seems to be responded to at the service level with dual stigma, increased bureaucracy, delays and less efficiency.

Lack of effective joint working

Parental substance misuse and mental ill health jointly highlight and are affected by the gaps between adults' and children's services and more generally in interagency working, with services often failing to coordinate an effective response to multiple issues within one family.

There are a number of reasons for the lack of an effective joined-up response to family needs by services. The Social Care Institute for Excellence (SCIE) in its report *Alcohol, Drug and Mental Health Problems: Working with Families* (Kearney *et al.* 2003a) identified the following causes/reasons for a lack of integrated responses.

- Discussion and clarification between agencies with different remits about their methods, terms of reference, values and priorities are needed if agencies are to fully understand one another and complement what each other do. However, this level of ongoing communication and relationship building is time consuming and this can be prohibitive. Also, such differences can lead to misunderstandings and tensions and sometimes to a resulting lack of motivation to work more closely together.

- When policies and procedures only focus on single users and fail to cater for multiple areas of need within the same individual or family, this can hinder, or at least fail to support, an integrated response.

Financial constraints and high eligibility thresholds

All agencies are operating within ever increasing budgetary constraints and the need to stretch limited resources leads to increasingly tighter 'gatekeeping' measures, such as eligibility thresholds that limit those who can access a particular service to those with the perceived highest need. In the mental health field, for example, this often means that mental health difficulties need to be regarded as 'severe and enduring' before a service user can access a service. In children and families statutory social work teams, the level of need encountered by a child often has to be quite high in many teams, increasingly with them being 'in need of protection' before assessments are undertaken. Further to this, the current financial climate has resulted in a reduction in capacity generally and in terms of implementing this and other service improvement agendas with specific grants being cut and redundancies in many organisations. The latter has led to many staff still in post having greater workloads and many conflicting demands on their time (SCIE 2012).

Another reason the SCIE review identified for a lack of effective joint working was that commissioning arrangements for smaller non-statutory agencies tended to be short term, with budgets only provided for a year or two at a time. Much time and energy is spent within such agencies trying to demonstrate the effectiveness of what they do in order to help secure the next round of funding. The consequence is that joint working arrangements are not as well developed as they could be.

Lack of a whole-family perspective in policy and performance indicators

Practitioners and managers working in the sites who worked intensively to try and implement the *Think Child, Think Parent, Think Family* guidance from SCIE (Diggins *et al.* 2011) reported that policies and performance indicators did not support their attempts to work together more effectively across adults' and children's services and this made progress more difficult (SCIE 2012). They reported that even where there was a commitment to doing this work in organisations, the sites found barriers to developing meaningful outcome indicators for families affected by parental mental ill health remained. However, Roscoe *et al.* in SCIE (2012) suggest that it is possible with an increased drive towards localism that the increased flexibility this brings to local regions to set their agendas could enable them to work on this more now. Martins (2013) also makes the point that payment-by-results models of drug and alcohol treatment providers may incentivise an increased implementation of outcome-based reform. However, to make a difference here, those outcomes need to include a family perspective. Further to this, Martins makes the point that if local strategies don't recognise the extent to which parental substance misuse can hinder good outcomes for children and their families, it may not be incorporated into Troubled Families programmes and priorities.

Lack of data collection

The data collection systems currently being operated do not measure and capture the size of the problem effectively, if at all. Until local statutory and voluntary agencies routinely and consistently have a record of how many parents and children are affected by parental mental health or substance misuse issues and what their presenting needs are, the recognition of the significance of these issues to services and the prioritisation of resources into these areas is unlikely to occur.

Lack of technical solutions

Some of the areas discussed above, such as effective joint working and helpful data collection are hindered by technical difficulties with services using different assessment and recording frameworks and incompatible IT systems. SCIE (2012) suggest this would most usefully be addressed at a national level.

A lack of accessible services

Fathers

Some of the tendency for services to fail to include or engage with fathers successfully (discussed earlier in relation to 'the practice level') occurs at a more strategic level. For example, it can be seen in part as being due to wider staffing and recruitment issues, as most of the workforce is female and such workforce issues need to be addressed. At the same time, more proactive steps can be taken to make the design of services more accessible and inclusive.

Men think 'Well this service isn't for me' so basically they don't have very high expectations of it. Wherever a service does engage fathers, they find that they are enthusiastic recipients of the service. Most men if you engage with them about parenting, will be so surprised that anyone is talking to them that they are grateful for anything. (National Voluntary Organisation in Department for Education and Skills 2006b, p.33)

Ghate, Shaw and Hazel (2000) examined some of the barriers that reduced fathers' likelihood of accessing Children's Centre and Sure Start programme-based support. Their feedback can be seen to be relevant to a far wider range of services. The barriers were listed as:

- policies and priorities that assume 'parents' to be synonymous with mothers
- referral systems that are geared towards mothers and children
- inconvenient opening hours
- lack of male staff and staff unsure how to interact with men due to being more used to women accessing the service
- 'feminised atmosphere'
- family centres perceived as a place of refuge for women
- women outnumbering men/lack of male presence
- some women were perceived as unfriendly, unwelcoming or even overtly hostile towards men
- activities – such as sitting drinking coffee, watching children play, talking with other parents, and aromatherapy – that were seen as 'female' and not enjoyed by men
- a perceived willingness in staff to engage with mothers as women as well as parents, but not fathers as men
- cultural ones, that is, some centres were offering services to Muslim women where including men would be inappropriate.

Another issue, identified earlier is the need to acknowledge situations where workers may be afraid of engaging with men whom they have come to perceive as hostile or even violent. A survey carried out with social workers by *Community Care* magazine found that many felt 'unprotected' and 'undermined' by their employers in relation to this issue and this directly affected their practice. Additionally, a lack of supervision and support systems to help workers deal with intimidation or threats of violence, along with a lack of support programmes for fathers, especially those who are violent, compounds failures to engage effectively with men in the circumstances (*Community Care* 2012).

Black and minority ethnic groups

There is strong evidence that black and minority ethnic (BME) groups receive fewer services or services that are of poorer quality and effectiveness than white service users. Research from the PricewaterhouseCoopers group, undertaken for the Department for Education and Skills (2006b) suggests that most local authorities are struggling to engage with BME groups effectively. They found BME parents showed increased reluctance to seek information and support through state services, had a greater fear of stigmatisation and were less likely to feel engaged with mainstream schools and services aimed at supporting parents. This was also borne out by Lavis (2014) in a Race Equality Foundation report that found young people from minority ethnic groups were less likely to access preventative mental health services.

Staff groups are rarely representative of the ethnic diversity of the communities they are based within and when there were black and minority ethnic staff, they were often informally placed in a role of being the 'BME specialist' and were poorly supported in this (Kurtz *et al.* 2005).

In relation to mental health specifically, the above findings were confirmed by SCIE's research briefing *Black and Minority Ethnic Parents with Mental Health Problems and their Children* (Greene, Pugh and Roberts 2008), which found that mental health problems among these groups, compounded by lack of adequate treatment responses and support, can have enduring adverse effects upon their children.

There is a large body of evidence of failures to provide equal access and opportunity to black and minority ethnic service users. In addition to there being inadequate treatment responses, *Delivering Race Equality: A Framework for Action* (Department of Health 2003) found there to be:

- reduced effectiveness of hospital treatment and longer hospital stays
- less likelihood of having broad needs addressed within treatment/care planning process
- more severe and coercive treatments
- lower access to talking treatments.

Similarly, the Care Quality Commission (2011) found people from BME communities were more likely to access mental health services through what Health Committee (2013 in Lavis 2014, p.6) called 'punitive or social control orientated gateways such as the prison service', were more likely to be admitted as inpatients and more likely to be detained under the Mental Health Act.

A *British Journal of Psychiatry* study (Leese *et al.* 2006) also found that black patients were likely to be younger on admission and to have had more previous hospital admissions, suggesting a pattern of 'revolving door contact' (Lyall 2006).

In relation to adults with substance misuse issues, there are some differences between different ethnic groups in both their patterns of drug use and the services they access. However, even with these differences taken into account, Abdulrahim (2006) reports that all BME groups are underrepresented within treatment services throughout the country and UK Drug Policy Commission (UKDPC) (2010a) also highlights the likelihood of underrepresentation.

Abdulrahim summarised the barriers to uptake of drug treatment by BME groups as being:

- a denial of drug use in some communities (by communities and professionals alike)
- a fear of confidentiality being breached
- the unrepresentative ethnicity of staff
- a lack of understanding by staff of cultural factors
- a lack of an appropriate service response
- an underdeveloped treatment for crack addiction
- a lack of service response to cannabis use
- drug treatments that tend to be more focused on opiate use than on other types of drug use
- a harm reduction strategy that focuses on injecting and is perceived by some to lack usefulness to non-injectors
- residential rehabilitation facilities that have often been found to be incapable of meeting diverse needs.

Further barriers to service take-up by adults from ethnic minority groups affected by either mental health or substance misuse issues are: that signposting information tends to be provided in English; most parenting programmes are evaluated with white and American samples; and no account is taken of potential differences in child-rearing and values (Department for Education and Skills 2006b).

There is a lack of research specifically into the experiences of BME children and young people affected by their parents' mental health or substance misuse (Adamson and Templeton 2012) but Lavis (2014) found children and young people were put off of accessing mental health services due to a lack of culturally appropriate services. Similarly, BME young carers are less likely to find services that meet their particular needs (Jones *et al.* 2002 in Parrott *et al.* 2008).

An illustration of the barriers to service take-up among young people can be found in the views obtained from them in a Young Minds study (Kurtz *et al.* 2005). These included:

- their previous experiences of discrimination and concerns about stigma
- their lack of a sense of inclusion in the local community
- the uncertain nature of the help they may have found, e.g. concerns about voluntary agencies closing due to lack of funds
- for those with uncertain legal status, how long they might be able to stay in the UK
- how to identify a mental health problem and what support would be available (felt by parents, too)

- 'going outside the family' to get help
- there being no interpreters available if they 'dropped in' for on-the-spot help
- staff in all services who had a poor awareness of their needs – conversely, young people greatly appreciated it when they found themselves 'finally understood' in specialist services
- a lack of choice in key members of staff, in terms of gender and cultural background, and a lack of younger staff from BME groups
- staff not always fully understanding the strong influence of parents' and communities' views and those of peer groups on the young people.

Malek (2011) argues that young people need to trust services before they will feel safe and confident enough to talk openly about their problems, and this is likely to be enhanced by practitioners showing a greater awareness of and interest in religious and cultural issues affecting them.

On a broader scale, there is a need for commissioners and service planners to obtain more data (that is meaningful) to better tailor commissioning plans and provision to the needs of BME children and their families and not to treat them as a homogenous group (Department of Health 2012).

This chapter has examined to some degree those things that get in the way of effective practice. Such barriers occur at many levels and range from longstanding, wider, societal issues, such as stigma, through more administrative and structural constraints, such as the design of policy and services, as well as critical issues of professional knowledge, values and skills. Thorough understanding of these barriers and their impacts can be a helpful precursor to identifying likely solutions for dealing with them.

5
How can services support families: approaches to assessment and intervention

This chapter discusses some of the key factors in improving the effectiveness of support to families so as to enhance their, and their children's, resilience. It highlights approaches to overcoming the barriers to effective practice. It discusses approaches to assessments and the principles and factors underpinning them and explores some of the factors that parents and children say are important for making services as useful and relevant to them as possible.

It considers a range of approaches with the potential to enhance practice and uses 'practice examples' to illustrate how services are trying to respond practically and positively to address critical issues in assessment and intervention.

Early intervention

It seems logical that the earlier people receive support, the more likely they are to overcome their difficulties. Better still, when difficulties seem likely to occur, the provision of services, support or the adoption of positive coping strategies can prevent problems arising, or at least from becoming overwhelming or entrenched. The case for early intervention and preventative practice is very strong, both morally and politically.

Current policy drivers in all the relevant service areas point strongly towards early intervention as a priority in the future shape of services.

Practice example 1 is an example of how services in Brighton collaborated to produce a resource for secondary schools and provide support to enable appropriate early responses to young people affected by parental substance misuse.

Practice example 1: The Hidden Ones, Brighton and Hove

In 2006 a collaboration between Brighton and Hove Healthy Schools Team, Brighton Oasis Project and Young Carers Project produced a communication resource.

This resource takes the form of a communication pack. It comprises a range of information for secondary schools to use in conjunction with local agencies to support individual students in situations where parental substance misuse has been identified. The pack includes:

- guidance for schools on how to respond to children and young people identified as vulnerable because of parental substance misuse
- information to support an enhanced school policy in respect of children affected by parental substance misuse
- information on available support within secondary schools and within outside local agencies
- case study material to support appropriate practice responses to children and young people.

Young Oasis – a service for 5–18-year-olds

Young Oasis[1] is a service for children and young people affected by familial substance misuse and is based within the Brighton Oasis Project. It is a voluntary-sector, substance-misuse service committed to preventing drug-related harm to women and children. Young Oasis offers a variety of creative therapeutic interventions for children and young people affected by familial drug or alcohol misuse. These range from weekly one-to-one therapy sessions with a creative therapist, to a Young Women's Creative Therapy Group run by qualified therapists in 12-week blocks, to holiday art groups during the school holidays with experienced group facilitators. Young Oasis has also been delivering an outreach group-work model within the local community. Children and young people are offered a First Meeting; from this consultation support is offered to suit an individual's needs.

---

1   For further information, contact: Jo Parker, 'Young Oasis', Brighton Oasis Project, 11 Richmond Place, Brighton BN2 9NA, Tel: 01273 696970 ext 203 or 0755 3360368.

Key factors in promoting early intervention are accessible services with clear referral pathways and useful, relevant information provided to potential users and referrers in locations where they are likely to access it. An agency seen to be promoting awareness and reducing stigma for people with mental health problems or substance misuse issues could actively reach many potential service users who otherwise might have a negative view of the service. Also, making information about possible support services more readily available may mean more people, who might not otherwise have thought of or known about what might help them, accessing them earlier and probably gaining more from them than if referred when their problems are more extreme.

> One of the difficulties you'll have…is measuring demand because demand isn't always expressed in terms of 'I want this' because there isn't a sense of entitlement. People don't always ask for what they want because they don't know they could have it. (National Voluntary Organisation in Department for Education and Skills 2006b, p.33)

Practice example 2 shows how a group parenting programme engages and supports women with mental health problems who have babies or young children.

Practice example 2: Mellow Parenting programme

The Mellow Parenting programme[2] combines support for parents as individuals with direct work to improve their relationship with their children. It developed from a concern that the parents most in need of help were least likely to engage with available support; that is the parents who were young, experiencing poor mental health and had additional health and social care needs. The Mellow Parenting programmes have a good track record in engaging with seldom reached parents. The high attendance rate (80% of parents attend 80% of the sessions) and good outcomes are due to a number of factors; the facilitators go the extra mile to remove barriers to joining the group, including providing transport and childcare through a children's group. There is respect for the individual and each parent and child is valued and nurtured. Time is taken to create safety in the groups so that parents can learn and grow. Solutions are not prescribed and the support of the group is used to create a sense of empowerment. Parents are invited to find new ways of interacting with their children by emphasising the positives whilst acknowledging difficulties.

Outcomes from attending a mellow parenting group include reductions in parental anxiety and depression, improvement in self-esteem and self-confidence, and a reduction in child behaviour problems. Children also had improved language skills and were therefore more likely to be ready for school.

As an example, one group member was a single mother in her twenties with two children who were looked-after and accommodated with a kinship carer due to parental neglect. She was homeless and was misusing alcohol. The woman had

---

2   For further information email: info@mellowparenting.org

very poor literacy skills having dropped out of school early. She had experienced a traumatic childhood; her father was an alcoholic, her mother was harsh and physically and emotionally abusive.

The young woman attended the group and barely missed a session. She began attending Alcoholics Anonymous (AA) and asked to be rehoused. By the end of the 14 weeks she had her children back living with her under a Supervision Order. She had also begun to volunteer at the family centre where the group was held and was running a cookery club at the local play scheme. These changes in her life were maintained over time. Mellow Parenting has a number of programmes available for all client groups including Mellow Bumps antenatal programme, Mellow Mums, Mellow Dads, Mellow Futures for parents with a learning disability and Mellow Ready for young care leavers.

Voluntary and compulsory support

Voluntary support is far more acceptable to families than compulsory intervention and is more likely to lead to better outcomes. At the lower tiers of need, self-referrals are more likely, whereas at the higher tiers there are more professional referrals. Support at the higher tiers is more likely to involve a degree of compulsion, because by the time needs have reached this level adverse impacts on children are so great that they have to be addressed. Compulsory interventions can still be effective, but close attention needs to be paid to helping people utilise and manage their experience of such interventions. Examples of this help include the following.

- Where parents are instructed to go on parenting courses – this is more likely to be effective if additional work takes place in advance of the courses to prepare parents for the group setting and ensure they are able to engage constructively and, not least, won't disrupt the group. Evidence suggests that such parents benefit from being mixed with parents who are receiving the support voluntarily (Department for Education and Skills 2006b).

- Where parents are referred for specialist assessments and interventions such as residential assessments – again, adequate preparation for the experience and a view that there is real potential for it to be effective, rather than being 'a safe place to fail' (Hart and Powell 2006), can lead to more positive outcomes.

- Where care proceedings have been initiated – in cases where parental substance misuse is a key element and a Family Drug and Alcohol Court (FDAC) is in operation in that area, a specialist multidisciplinary team of practitioners can assess, devise and coordinate an intervention with the family.

Practice example 3 describes the FDAC and shows a different approach to care proceedings with an emphasis on problem-solving and direct work with families during the process.

Practice example 3: Family Drug and Alcohol Court (FDAC): a different approach to care proceedings

Launched in January 2008, the FDAC is a new way of dealing with care proceedings when parental substance misuse causes harm to children.

The pilot (2008–2012) was funded by the Department for Education, the Ministry of Justice, the Home Office, the Department of Health and three inner-London local authorities (Camden, Islington, and Westminster). Since April 2012, when government funding came to an end, the FDAC specialist team has been funded by a consortium of five London authorities, including Southwark, and Hammersmith and Fulham, as well as the original three.

The intervention

FDAC is a specialist, problem-solving court operating within the framework of care proceedings, with parents given the choice to choose between this and the usual approach. Working with the court is a specialist multidisciplinary team of practitioners provided by a partnership between the Tavistock and Portman NHS Foundation Trust and the children's charity, Coram. The team: carries out assessments; devises and coordinates an individual intervention plan; helps parents engage and stay engaged with substance misuse and parenting services; carries out direct work with parents; gets feedback on parental progress from services; and provides regular reports on parental progress to the court and to all others involved in the case. Attached to the team are volunteer parent mentors to provide support to parents.

The aim of the FDAC is to help parents stabilise/stop using drugs/alcohol and, where possible, to keep families together. Instead of a normal care proceedings court process, a family chosen for the FDAC process will go through a slightly different process, with more regular court hearings with the same judge for the whole process. Cases in FDAC are heard by two dedicated district judges, with two further district judges available to provide backup for sickness and holidays. Cases are dealt with by the same judge throughout. Guardians are appointed to FDAC cases immediately. Legal representatives attend the first two court hearings, but thereafter there are regular, fortnightly court reviews that legal representatives do not attend unless there is a particular issue requiring their input.

The court reviews are the problem-solving, therapeutic aspect of the court process. They provide opportunities for regular monitoring of parents' progress and for judges to engage and motivate parents, to speak directly to parents and social workers and to find ways of resolving problems that may have arisen.

Like any care proceedings, there is still a potential for the family to lose their children, but the FDAC process has been set up to encourage success and to be as supportive as possible. They are given time and support to think about the process, what's on offer and to come to a decision about participating. They are encouraged to discuss it with their social workers and others in their networks and are not pressured to come to an immediate decision.

Impact

FDAC has been independently evaluated. The evaluation of the pilot was conducted by a research team at Brunel University and was funded by the Nuffield Foundation and the Home Office. The independent evaluation notes that FDAC is distinctive because it is a court-based family intervention that aims to improve children's outcomes by addressing the entrenched difficulties of their parents.

Key findings

- More FDAC parents controlled their substance misuse and there was a higher rate of reunification with their children than those going through usual proceedings.

- FDAC parents were offered more help than comparison parents for their substance misuse problems. FDAC played a significant role in this, as it coordinated access to other community services. They accessed substance misuse services quicker, received a broader range of services in the first six months and were more successful at staying in treatment throughout the proceedings. More FDAC parents received help from housing, benefits and domestic violence services.

- Parents interviewed at either stage of the evaluation shared the same positive views including saying they would recommend FDAC to other parents.

- Parents with previous experience of care proceedings found FDAC to be a more helpful court process – one that gave them a fair chance to change their lifestyle and parent their child well.

Quotes from those involved in FDAC

FDAC has helped me be the sort of person I want to be. It's helped me remain focused and motivated and instilled in me a real sense of achievement and confidence. (Parent)

FDAC have good links with substance misuse services. For cases not in FDAC it's very hard to get information from substance misuse services whereas in FDAC the services are there and there's discussion with them at the IPM (Intervention Planning Method. (Social worker)

Clients in FDAC feel, not exactly relaxed, but they seem to take on board things a little bit more. They seem to understand a bit better why they are doing something and they are happier with the process, even if it is not something they want. (Adult treatment service)

This court is different. We don't do conflict. We minimise hostility. This is about solving problems. (Judge)

Instead of fibbing we're encouraged to be honest and if we relapse, or lapse even, we're told it wouldn't be the end of it, because they would work with us about that. They were being honest with us and making it easier for us to be honest with them. (Parent)

There will be times when compulsory intervention will mean children being removed permanently from their families because it has not been possible to ensure their safety at home. And sometimes this is for the best. Adoption and fostering can work well for some children. Forrester and Harwin (2006) found, in their study of cases within four London boroughs over two years, that many of the children who had been fostered or adopted in that time were showing better outcomes than those with similar family circumstances and experiences who were still at home.

However, even when such concrete and seemingly 'final decisions' have been made, such as applying for a care order and adoption, the needs of the family still need to be addressed. The impact on family members of what they have been through, the changes, transitions and arrangements for them to continue to see each other or to make sense of what has happened, need careful considered support.

Approaches to assessment

Most of the professionals reading this handbook are involved to some extent in undertaking assessments within their services, whether assessing potential users for eligibility for their service, undertaking an Early Help assessment, tailoring the service appropriately or by being a member of a team around the family or a partner in a wider professional network and contributing through meetings, discussions and reports to an assessment being coordinated by someone else. Others work within lead agencies carrying out a formal assessment, such as a mental health assessment or an assessment under the *Framework for the Assessment of Children in Need and their Families* (Department of Health 2000). The application of this framework for assessing children's needs and factors that affect them within three domains – family and environmental factors, parenting capacity and the child's developmental needs – and critically the interaction between them, was explored in greater depth in Chapter 2.

More recently, the implementation of the *Common Assessment Framework* following the Children Act 2004 means that an even greater variety of relevant professionals are involved in assessments. Assessments should always be based on clear and rigorous analysis of information about the family in a way that makes the process transparent and explicable to a broad audience. The issue of analysis within assessments is a much discussed and important one though it is not an altogether straightforward process, since weighing up complex issues necessarily involves deploying and melding analytical and intuitive processes, skills and knowledge within an ever-changing and complex social, cultural and political context.

How practitioners could be supported in improving the analytical element of assessment by introducing different tools and approaches is described in greater detail in Dalzell and Sawyer (2011, 2016), but some of the points from their text are highlighted below.

Assessment as intervention

There is a thin line between assessment and intervention and the distinction can be false or over-simplistic. However, practitioners have to exercise high-level skills and judgement to ensure that assessments are not simply about matching service users to services, gatekeeping resources or investigating deficits in family functioning. Done well, assessments can and should increase service users' self-knowledge and improve their desire to make changes, and they should be family friendly. Also, when undertaken reflectively, assessments should lead to professionals identifying their own needs for additional skills or training and, through identifying and recording any unmet service user needs, helping agencies to learn about the need for the creation of additional services and opportunities (Hamer 2005).

There is a particular challenge for those undertaking child protection investigations or assessments to engage families in the process in a way that is beneficial to them. If some level of partnership or collaboration between worker and service user can be established early on, this can make a major difference to the direction that the work takes later on and in turn the outcomes for the children and the family. Turnell and Edwards (1999) argue that even child protection investigations can be therapeutic, in that they can help develop a family's understanding of the issues affecting them and offer support and education, with interventions being 'the icing on the cake'. They see the relationship between professional and service user as having the potential to be the principal vehicle for change. Recognition of how crucial this engagement and direct work is to effective practice was recently reinforced by this observation from Ofsted inspections:

> What is striking in the local authorities judged to be 'good', is the centrality and importance of direct work with families. They report having stable relationships with social workers and there is consistent case file evidence showing that assessment is derived from on-going and regular contact housed in a relationship that is firmly established between the worker and the family. This contrasts directly with weaker practice, where assessment is conducted as a single exercise dominated by forms. (Ofsted 2014, p.6)

Values and reflexivity

It is essential that those undertaking assessments are able to recognise the impact of their feelings and values on their assessment and interactions with families.

Forrester (2004) and Galvani and Forrester (2010) stress the importance of this in relation to substance misuse because it is such a value-laden subject. All individual professionals will have some preconceptions, concerns, stereotypes or experience (personal or professional) of substance or alcohol use that affect their responses to it. Preconceptions could influence one in favour of either over-zealous interventions or naïve and over-optimistic inaction. This can also be said of mental ill health, where there are the dangers of overreacting due to fear and misunderstanding, reinforced by frequent media portrayal of 'dangerousness'. Conversely, feeling great sympathy for people in distress and wanting to help or prove to them that you are not there to make things worse can make it harder to respond quickly and appropriately if they are becoming unable to meet their children's needs.

In social research, a 'cultural review' checklist is sometimes used (devised by McCracken (1988)) at the outset of the work as a way of triggering an examination of cultural assumptions. Holland (2004) adapted the original checklist for social work use. Undertaking the review involves asking oneself questions at the outset of work or on receipt of referral information, such as the following.

- What do I know about individuals with these life experiences?
- Where does my knowledge come from?
- What prejudices may I hold (positive or negative)?
- What might surprise me and why would it be a surprise?
- How might I/the assessment and my agency be perceived by this family?
- What agency norms and practices do I take with me on an assessment (e.g. awareness of risk, thresholds of 'good-enough parenting', resource restrictions)?

This approach helps bring preconceived ideas or values into consciousness in order to help minimise their potential adverse impact on the integrity of an assessment.

Hypothesising

The tendency for first impressions to last and for human beings to seek out and notice information that supports their original ideas has been long observed and well documented (Scott 1998; Sheldon 1987). Information that is contrary to strongly held views or ideas is more easily dismissed or even goes unnoticed as information is sought to confirm our biases, a phenomenon now well known and widely accepted as a major challenge in assessments.

One of the most common, problematic tendencies in human cognition…is our failure to review judgements and plans – once we have formed a view on what is going on, we often fail to notice or to dismiss evidence that challenges that picture. (Fish, Munro and Bairstow 2008, p.9)

Once again, social research methods can assist here. Holland (2004) discusses the importance of 'hypothesising' at the outset and (at staged intervals) throughout assessments. A hypothesis is a proposed explanation for something; so in a family support context, a hypothesis is a way of understanding a family situation. For example, if a child is frequently late for school or is increasingly tired and withdrawn there could be a range of reasons for this, including the following.

- It may be a result of increased parental stress whereby the child is not receiving the usual level of support with getting up and ready for school.
- It could be that the child is anxious about a school matter.
- It could be they are worried about a move to secondary school and not sleeping as a result.
- The child may have a substance misuse problem.

The presence of different factors (known about by professionals) will all influence which hypothesis or hypotheses are held at different stages.

This process of generating ideas about family situations usually occurs almost naturally. However, if left at this, the chances are that only two or three ideas will be generated and the natural human tendency to find information that supports these ideas will kick in. Raynes (in Calder and Hackett 2003) suggests the need to generate as many hypotheses early on as possible and Holland (2004) suggests then actively seeking to disprove each one, identifying information that confirms or disproves them until one or two strong explanations emerge that are well supported. In reaching best judgements on the information thus gathered, it is important that professionals continually reflect on and continually challenge their assumptions and analyses. In *Ten Pitfalls and How to Avoid Them: What Research Tells Us* Broadhurst *et al.* (2010) suggest questions practitioners and managers should ask themselves to guard against this confirmation bias. Questions for practitioners include the following.

- Am I remaining curious and inquisitive about what I am seeing and assessing?
- Am I open to new information?
- Would I be prepared to change my mind about this case?
- How confident am I that I have sufficient information upon which to base my judgements?
- Do I need to add a 'health warning' about the strength of evidence contained in this assessment and the implications for decision-making?

Needs and outcomes focus

Assessments are most likely to be helpful if they are focused on needs and outcomes, a very easy stance to agree with in principle but which can prove to be something of a struggle in practice. One of the main barriers is the tendency to jump to considering services too early on. A helpful brake on this might be to consider the response/responses to the question 'What might be the needs for this child/family?' If the response includes things such as:

- speech therapy
- further assessment by (some specialist agency)
- counselling
- behavioural management support or respite care

then the question has not been answered. These are all services and, whilst telling us what possible options there are for meeting needs, the actual needs are still unknown.

By stepping back and considering what the needs might be (that the above options could possibly meet), we may come up with some of the following.

- The child needs to develop their verbal or communication skills to enable them to interact more with their peers.
- A parent needs support in addressing their alcohol dependence.
- A parent needs help in stabilising their severe mood swings or anxiety.
- An adolescent needs support with a bereavement.
- A parent needs help in setting boundaries for their child.
- A parent needs a break from caring for their disabled child so that they can give some one-to-one attention to their non-disabled child.

It is this latter list of needs that should be the starting point, with services being considered later down the line.

Once the needs of family members are identified, then 'outcomes' can be considered. We can ask: if the child's need were met, how would we know? What would this look like? It may be thought that if the child starts speaking more in class and interacting more confidently with their peers, we can see that as a concrete outcome of the need being met. Only then, when we have identified needs and what the outcome of them being met would look like, is it appropriate to consider what things might individually or collectively help move towards that outcome.

There is usually more than one approach to meeting the same need. If needs are the starting point for intervention rather than services, then if one service makes a family wary or adds to their stress, another form of intervention can be considered that may be more acceptable and useful to the family. This approach fits well with the use of the *Common Assessment Framework* and the *Framework for the Assessment of Children in Need and their Families* (Department of Health 2000) and is discussed more fully in Dalzell and Sawyer (2011, 2016 forthcoming).

Assessing resilience

A helpful framework for assessment where parents have mental health and substance misuse problems, given the multifaceted nature of these difficulties, is the resilience/vulnerability matrix. It provides a framework for weighing up factors that create adversity in children's lives and increase their vulnerability alongside those factors that research has shown can contribute to increased resilience.

Using the resilience/vulnerability matrix

Completion of the matrix requires the practitioner to have a working knowledge of resilience theory and the factors that contribute to the different axes of the matrix. A good starting point would be to read Chapters 3, 4 and 5 of Daniel *et al.* (2010) *Child Development for Child Care and Protection Workers.*

Sufficient information will need to have been accumulated from assessment or other interaction with a child and their carers, family and involved professionals. Each axis of the matrix contains a scale from 0 to 10, with 0 being an absence of factors contributing to that domain of the matrix and 10 being the highest incidence of contributory factors.

Although the original model of the risk and resilience matrix which appeared in the 1999 publication referred to above does not include any scaling of the various factors, we have included it in this adapted model because we know from experience that most social work practitioners and child care professionals are very familiar with the idea of scaling. Please note:

- Scaling in the context is not intended to be a scientific exercise but completed in the same spirit as in, for example, practice approaches such as Solution Focussed working/ Signs of Safety and Motivational Interviewing.

- In this context, the professional and or the family member /young person is invited to scale the factors to reflect their own weighting of the level of concern, thus providing a starting point for reflection and discussion and a benchmark to move on from. This encourages critical thinking and discussion rather than suggesting that there is some scientific answer based on the numbers.

- The completed matrix creates a visual map to refer to now and in the future in terms of mapping changes and developments and to help in assessing the impact of interventions.

Taking each axis in turn, the information that has been gathered is scored on the 0–10 scale. For example, for a child with a secure attachment and good problem-solving skills, who is popular with peers, has a high IQ and is doing well at school, this would most likely lead to a high score on the *resilience* axis of the matrix. If, however, that child has been self-harming for some time and this is becoming more severe over time, and they are developing anxiety problems that are interfering with their day-to-day life, a score to reflect this would be placed on the *vulnerability* axis. If the same young person is living in a family situation with domestic abuse, parental mental ill health and financial insecurity, this would indicate a significant score on the *adversity* axis, but if they also have good relationships with teachers and other adults and made good use of support and advice offered from the school counsellor, this would be noted on the *protective environment* axis. The matrix is most useful when used as an interactive tool with children and young people as active agents in the process.

There are no right and wrong answers and the scoring will be a matter of professional judgement. Indeed, whenever we use this tool in training there are vigorous debates as to the impact – harmful or beneficial – of various factors in children's lives. The completion of the matrix only represents the understanding of the child's situation at that time and by those involved in constructing it. It will be informed by theory, research, practice wisdom, local knowledge and information gleaned from a range of sources, including the child themselves.

The process of considering and plotting the information is in itself a useful process and requires thoughtfulness and possibly debate if being done with others, but there is another stage that can create a powerful visual map. Once all of the axes have been considered and plotted, the points can be joined with a drawn line to create a shape that will be spread across the four domains (located more within some than others). This visual map can help in assessment and planning by providing a snapshot, but can also be useful for recording progress if completed at various intervals.

Where the shape sits predominantly in the top right-hand quadrant of the two axes, this suggests that the child is both resilient and protected and more likely to be able to recover from any difficulties they face. This is the safest area for children to be and universal services can support and build on these positive factors.

Where the shape sits predominantly in the lower right quadrant, this indicates that the child is protected, but for whatever reason also vulnerable. This will mean that the planning for this child should focus on maintaining the support whilst building up their resilience.

Where the shape sits predominantly in the top left quadrant, this indicates a child who exhibits signs of resilience whilst remaining in adverse circumstances. These are the children who targeted and specialist services should be working with to increase the level of protection, in partnership with the child and their family, whether by raising them from poverty or taking action to safeguard against abuse. One criticism of this model is that resilient children in risky situations may be ignored as relatively safe. It is crucial to recognise that no matter how resilient children may be, there will be times when the risks are too severe to ignore, and the presence of resilience factors should never be an excuse for lack of attention or inaction.

If the shape sits predominantly in the lower left corner of the graph, it indicates the most vulnerable child who does not have resilience or factors within their environment to provide protection. This child will need intensive specialist intervention. As well as identifying the associated risk, this model allows us to develop care plans in two directions – to increase the level of protection and to improve children's resilience, improving the chances of reducing risk.

Figure 5.1: Resilience/vulnerability matrix

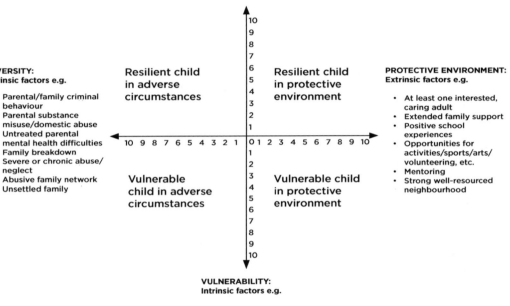

RESILIENCE:
Intrinsic factors e.g.

- Secure attachment
- High self-esteem
- Sociability/friendships
- Empathy for self and others
- High IQ
- Talents and interests
- Flexible temperament
- Problem-solving skills
- Attractive

ADVERSITY:
Extrinsic factors e.g.

- Parental/family criminal behaviour
- Parental substance misuse/domestic abuse
- Untreated parental mental health difficulties
- Family breakdown
- Severe or chronic abuse/neglect
- Abusive family network
- Unsettled family

Resilient child in adverse circumstances

Resilient child in protective environment

Vulnerable child in adverse circumstances

Vulnerable child in protective environment

PROTECTIVE ENVIRONMENT:
Extrinsic factors e.g.

- At least one interested, caring adult
- Extended family support
- Positive school experiences
- Opportunities for activities/sports/arts/volunteering, etc.
- Mentoring
- Strong well-resourced neighbourhood

VULNERABILITY:
Intrinsic factors e.g.

- Insecure attachment[s]
- Minority status
- Infant
- Poor educational attainment
- Disability/communication differences
- A loner/no friends
- Few interests
- Lack of empathy towards self and others
- Poor self-care
- Institutional care
- Unresolved losses

Adapted and developed from an original model in Daniel
et al. (1999) *Child Development for Child Care and Child
Protection Workers.* London: Jessica Kingsley Publishers.

Representing children's views and needs in assessments

Some professionals who work directly with children as a matter of course, providing specialist or universal services directly to them, are particularly skilled in recognising and describing children's needs and feelings. Others, for example, those whose role is wider – either working with whole families or with individual parents or carers – may need support in interpreting or understanding children's experiences.

For those professionals such as social workers who need to try and establish children's needs, views and wishes, they will need to take individualised, flexible and creative approaches to maximising children's and young people's opportunities to be consulted meaningfully. They may also find consulting with a range of people who know the child, observing the child in a range of settings and finding out about others' observations in a variety of settings over time, helpful. Disabled children's views and perspectives are particularly poorly represented in assessments, as practitioners often lack the confidence, skills and creativity to access their feelings and views. Drawing on all possible resources and creative communication techniques and using equipment or facilitators where appropriate, in addition to allowing sufficient time to enable children to contribute to assessment, are essential.

In reality, the information and knowledge about children's views and wishes will often be partial, so it is important to acknowledge gaps and limitations in our understanding so that we don't misrepresent children through assumptions or partial information.

Assessments need to keep the child at the centre and should seek to understand how the child sees and experiences their situation. This will involve asking questions about 'what life is like:

- when they wake up?
- when they go to bed?
- when parents are intoxicated or withdrawing?
- what are their hopes and fears?
- who can they turn to?'

(Hart and Powell 2006)

This will involve working with children in a way which 'rather than putting them on the spot...enables them to tell a story' (Kroll and Taylor 2003, p.267) and workers considering not only the child's current experience but also their experience in the past months as well as what they are likely to experience in the future.

Bringing fathers/significant males into focus

The critical importance of including fathers and other significant males in work with families and the deficiencies in practice when such a focus is lacking were discussed in Chapter 4. Recognition and concern about the lack of focus on fathers – both potential risks and protections – has seen development of new information and resources directed at practitioners, by the NSPCC, *Community Care* and the Fatherhood Institute among others. Some common messages that have emerged include: the need to make explicit from the outset the father's crucial role, making a determined effort to involve fathers, including making arrangements that are practical and convenient for them, and involving them in assessments. In their recent 'top tips for social workers' in engaging fathers, *Community Care* suggests that social workers: 'research theories of masculinity to try and understand the motivations of men involved in a case' and that: 'men are more powerfully motivated by the desire to be a good father than by the effect of their behaviour on women' so: 'a good starting point is to ask them: "what does it mean to be a good father?"'(*Community Care* 2012). New developments to aid practice include a bank of resources developed by the Fatherhood Institute, which includes a good practice guide jointly developed with Family Rights Group, *Engaging with Men in social Care: A Good Practice Guide* (Fatherhood Institute 2013). This guide, derived from a 2011–13 project run jointly by the two organisations, suggests strategies for engaging with men in, or attached to, families in which a child is at risk or may become so. They point out that professionals are more likely to be successful in engaging fathers when they:

- present the father's engagement as expected and important from the start
- proactively seek out the men and acknowledge their role as parent or carer and their expert knowledge about and concern for their child and family
- engage with men's versions of events in an open and exploratory way, and don't assume that he is 'the problem' without adequate evidence
- engage informally with individual fathers before proposing ongoing intervention
- follow up those fathers who don't participate
- emphasise repeatedly the benefits to the child of their father's participation
- assess routinely fathers' needs, including their mental health
- engage with fathers who don't live with their children
- encourage mothers, children and other family members to think about fathers' importance and help to involve them.

Thinking 'whole family'

The need for assessments to focus on wider family and social networks is well recognised and generally accepted; realising this in practice, however, continues to be a considerable challenge. As discussed above, a whole-family approach requires proactive efforts by service providers to engage fathers as well as mothers and in particular such an approach recognises the importance to children of fathers who live separately from, but still have contact with, them. Additionally, families welcome services that are inclusive of fathers in their approach (Kroll and Taylor 2003).

There also needs to be more attention paid to both the needs of extended family members and the potential contribution to assessments and support that they can make.

When relatives are significantly involved in supporting families, professionals should avoid making assumptions that they are 'coping' (Hart and Powell 2006). It can be particularly difficult for wider family members to bring up their own support needs, which can arise from the practicalities of providing support, the emotional toll of worrying about their family members, divided loyalties, guilt and conflicts. Relatives may also need support and information to help them understand mental health needs or substance issues.

Similarly, kinship carers, known to play a significant role in families affected by parental mental health and/or substance misuse difficulties, often experience conflicting loyalties, anger and worry about the parents and guilt about their own role and responsibility in the parents' problems. The support they receive can be patchy or entirely lacking. To be effective in identifying and meeting children's needs, assessments and interventions must pay critical attention to the roles and needs of kinship carers.

Placing knowledge in context

The information available to those carrying out assessments will usually be partial, hence the importance of putting knowledge and information into context within assessment reports or when communicating about the family situation. Assessments can sometimes be over-reliant on short-term observations, focusing on acute episodes rather than reflecting the ebbs and flows of everyday life (Aldridge 1999). Clearly identifying the extent of knowledge of the family that is available, and being explicit about gaps in knowledge, is the only way to reduce the misrepresentation that can occur.

Also, showing awareness and sensitivity about the stress generated by the assessment process itself (or by the search for support or even receiving the support itself), will help place family reactions to this stress into context. Turnell and Edwards (1999) give the following example to illustrate this. If a parent leaves a meeting early in frustration, they can all too easily be labelled uncooperative when in fact they had a terrible week, were being asked questions they had been asked before and thought that professionals had already made up their minds.

Turnell and Edwards stress the need to search for detail to explore all positive and negative factors from sources inside and outside the family. They argue that this will will make it more possible to identify the antecedents, to see patterns and to pick up on feelings and opportunities for change (Turnell and Edwards 1999).

Assessing the impact of specific issues

The points made so far about assessments in general apply to assessments of family members affected by parental mental health problems and/or substance misuse. All assessments should focus on the wide-ranging needs and experiences of families. However, whilst this broad focus is right and helpful, and indeed parents have often given feedback that they want professionals to see their lives as a whole and not to attribute all their difficulties to mental health or substance problems (Tunnard 2002a, 2004), there is still a need for close attention to issues such as the impact of substance use, mental health and domestic violence, especially when they occur together.

Assessment of risk and protective factors should be considered and mitigating support offered/action taken as appropriate. In the following two sections, some of the areas for specific consideration in these circumstances are highlighted.

When it comes to decision-making, the key questions that arise from the models that follow are: 'What needs to change to protect the child now or minimise the future impact of these problems on them?' and 'How can this be achieved within that child's timeframe?' In thinking about the latter, the professional needs to consider the questions.

- Can resilience factors be bolstered?
- Can risks be reduced through support to the family?
- What are the wishes and feelings of the child?
- What timescales are appropriate to the child's needs?
- Can the family make the necessary changes and can they be achieved within such timescales?
- How does the likelihood of plans succeeding weigh against the potential impact of failure?
- If a child cannot be cared for by their family how can future relationships be supported?

Substance misuse

A range of helpful models has been developed to assist practitioners in focusing their assessment of the impact of parental substance misuse on children.

For example Hart and Powell (2006) have devised a very helpful Model for Assessment of Parental Drug Use, which overlays the *Framework for the Assessment of Children in Need and their Families* with particular questions of pertinence for children of drug-using parents.

Short-term risks of immediate harm need to be assessed along with those of longer-term risks to give the cumulative impact on the child or young person's emotional and behavioural well-being. It is also essential to consider how other issues and factors that are present but not directly related to substance misuse (such as family conflict or a learning disability) are impacting on the child and affecting their circumstances.

Forrester (2004) puts forward the following Four Assessment Principles to assist in focusing assessments of children's needs when there is parental substance misuse.

Four assessment principles

1. Maintain a focus on the child. Collecting information on the pattern of drug use is of limited utility in making an assessment if all the other variables are not focused on. How does the substance use impact on the child? How is the child progressing and understanding any reasons for the difficulties they may have?

2. Adults' management of their own life can be a good indicator of their ability to look after a child (the measure being whether the parent is causing themselves harm through a failure to manage their own lives).

3. Past behaviour is the best predictor of future behaviour. A good chronology and full social history, which is best completed by involving the parent and young person (if appropriate), can greatly assist this.

4. A variety of sources should be used for information. This includes different agencies along with wider family, such as grandparents, as valuable sources of information and support.

    (Adapted from Donald Forrester's work in Phillips 2004, pp.172–4)

The model in Figure 5.2 utilises and adapts models produced by Forrester (2004) and Hart and Powell (2006) to highlight the risk and protective factors that need to be weighed up when considering the impact of substance misuse on children and their families.

Figure 5.2: Links in a chain

Parenting capacity – risks and concerns

Details of drug use

Previous parenting capacity concerns

Relationship/ partner reinforcing drug use?

Impact on parent's health/behaviour/mood

Impairment of caring ability or physical/ emotional availability to child

Prioritising drugs over child

Inconsistency/unreliable to child

Messages to child about drug use/ offending behaviour e.g. normalising

Family and environmental – risks and concerns

Offending behaviour and convictions

Lack of engagement now or previously with drug treatment

Isolation/ lack of support

Secrecy affecting relationships outside/ inside home

Inadequate material resources (money and housing)

Exposure to risky adults/activities in the home

Stigma/negative community attitudes

Child's developmental needs – risks and concerns

Effects of prenatal exposure to drugs

Special health needs as a result of the above

Access or exposure to drugs/ equipment

Negative impact on attachments and feeling valued

Effect on child's attitudes to drug use and offending behaviour that increase their vulnerability

Experience of loss or bereavement

Sibling drug use or impaired sibling relationships

Secrecy, stigma and social exclusion

Negative impact on friendships

Caring responsibilities

Long-term risks and concerns into adulthood

Previous risks/concerns not addressed or resolved

Unplanned/unsupported transitions

Lack of family support

Lack of professional support/timely interventions

Social isolation – no stable main relationship/ lack of friends

Unemployment

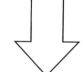

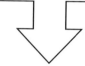

Impact of substance misuse on parenting capacity

Impact on child's development: daily experience

Likely future impact on child (and into adulthood)

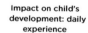

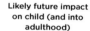

Parenting capacity – positives

Effective strategies to protect child from impact of drugs

Previous parenting capacity positive

Resilience factors

Parent/family non-substance misusing partner, use out of home, lack of violence

Social/environmental

Supportive wider family/ community

Resilience factors

Child experiencing success outside the home e.g. school

High intelligence, good coping strategies, exposure for shorter time

Social/environmental

Supportive school

Good relationship/s with adults outside family

Parent/Family

Good relationship with one parent

Resilience factors (that reduce chance of difficulties persisting into adulthood)

Child/young person

A planned transition to adulthood

Social/environmental

A good job, a good main relationship, good friends

Harbin and Murphy (2000) put forward the model in Figure 5.3. Where possible, this should be considered jointly by substance misuse and child and family practitioners so as to optimise the information available and the understanding of practitioners of the family circumstances.

The first stage involves gaining an understanding of the nature of substance use, including its impact on the lifestyle of the parent and their relationship to the substance or its 'meaning' for them. The second stage considers both the parent's own experience of being parented, their attitudes and expectations about their own parenting role and the impact of their substance use (or withdrawal) on their parenting. The third stage considers the impact these factors have on the child and any needs they have arising from this. The last stage involves consideration of the level of childcare demand on the parent, which will be influenced by the age, developmental stage and number of children, as well as the support available from other adults.

Figure 5.3: The assessment process

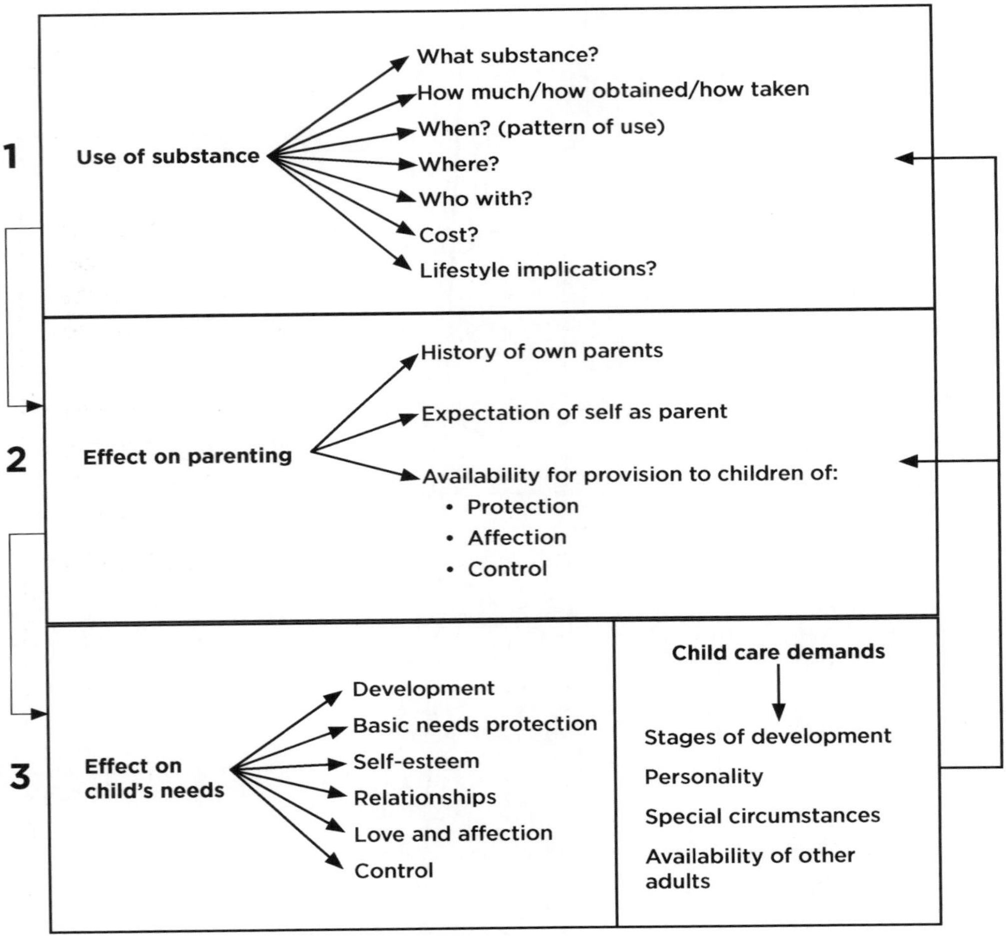

Additionally practitioners will need to have cognisance of other factors in operation. For example, the guilt, shame and remorse that many parents feel is hard to face (Kroll and Taylor 2003) and needs to be considered sensitively within the approach taken to assessment.

Many parents are strongly motivated by wanting to put things right for their children. Becoming a parent or realising the impact the addiction has on parenting can be strong motivators for change; as can, in some circumstances, the reality of children potentially being separated from parents (Bates *et al.* 1999). Assessments need to search for strengths and scope for change.

Mental health

In supporting families affected by parental mental health issues it is important to establish patterns that occur, in order to find ways of identifying early on when mental health is deteriorating or relapse is occurring. Establishing potential arrangements for early identification, ongoing monitoring and access to support and intervention when necessary is ideal but requires proactive and flexible services.

The following provides a list of dimensions to be explored in assessments of families affected by parental mental health problems. This is taken from Gopfert *et al.* (2004).

Dimensions of parenting formulation

Focus on the role of parent – this includes assessing parenting capacity in line with the Assessment Framework headings. It also includes considering whether the parent understands and has age-appropriate expectations of their child; the parent's ability to discuss their mental illness appropriately with their child; and any evidence of role reversal.

Focus on the role of child – this includes considering: the child's developmental needs within the Assessment Framework; their attachment status; any unusual, 'non-childlike' behaviour, including involvement in parent's symptoms or substance misuse and 'parentification'; and what protective factors are present.

Focus on the impact of mental illness on the role of parent – this includes considering the parent's:

- sense of responsibility for self, child and family
- capacity to acknowledge risks to child
- level of disturbance, instability and violent tendencies (impulse control)
- behaviour and psychiatric symptoms where they directly affect parenting capacity, including alcohol/substance misuse
- level of commitment to child
- motivation for change, including past history

- capacity to reflect
- attitude to social norms/relationship to society
- attitude to professionals; use of help and clinical interventions.

Focus on the role of 'well'/other parent (if relevant) – this includes considering the other parent's:

- commitment to maintaining the family or commitment to the relationship with the child
- capacity to be available/to intervene on the child's behalf, if and when necessary
- relationship to the child
- attitude to the illness of their partner
- health and emotional resources.

Focus on the role of spouse/partner (if relevant) – this includes considering the extent to which there is any:

- history of violence/spouse abuse
- capacity to work together as parents
- patterns, style and intensity of marital conflict
- ability to communicate.

Focus on the context and extended family – this includes considering the following factors:

- access to relationship with an adult who is committed to providing support and care for child and/or parent
- degree and patterns of support from extended family, directly to child as well as to parent
- parent's relationship to own parents
- quality of non-family network
- financial/housing status
- environmental stress/life events/current stressors.

Figure 5.4 is a reworked version of the model put forward in Hart and Powell (2006) for practitioners to use where children may be in need as a result of parental drug misuse. It is one that they had in turn adapted from the *Framework for the Assessment of Children in Need and their Families* (Department of Health 2000).

As highlighted in earlier chapters, most notably in Chapter 4, well-recognised challenges for professionals include undertaking assessments when there are complex issues such as parental mental health problems involved. While the needs and experiences of children and parents vary widely and while some children will do well and thrive, without the right support and intervention, the adverse impacts of these difficulties on children's outcomes can be significant and long-lasting.

The adapted framework tries to support practitioners to address some of the known barriers to practice such as a:

- lack of knowledge and confidence about adult mental health issues
- risk of becoming too focused on parents' concerns and problems
- complex array of single-user services and lack of cross-agency working
- lack of focus on the whole family and wider networks.

The issues highlighted within the three domains are not exhaustive and the model should be used as a prompt to guide thinking and discussion and not as a checklist. It is not expected that an individual practitioner would hold all the necessary knowledge but that they collaborate and co-work with colleagues within and across agencies.

Figure 5.4: Adapted Assessment framework for use with families where there are parental mental health problems

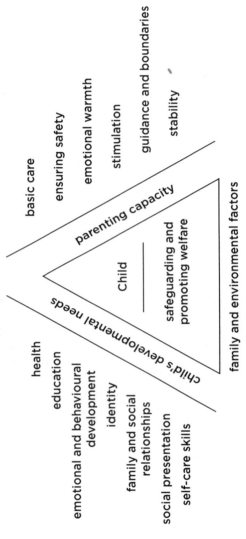

CHILD'S DEVELOPMENTAL NEEDS (left side of triangle):
- health
- education
- emotional and behavioural development
- identity
- family and social relationships
- social presentation
- self-care skills

PARENTING CAPACITY (right side of triangle):
- basic care
- ensuring safety
- emotional warmth
- stimulation
- guidance and boundaries
- stability

FAMILY AND ENVIRONMENTAL FACTORS (bottom of triangle):
- family history and functioning
- wider family
- housing
- employment
- income
- family's social integration
- community resources

Centre of triangle: Child — safeguarding and promoting welfare

Top right box (Parenting capacity):
- » Details of mental health problems and impact on parental health behaviour/mood
- » Details of treatments, interventions and attitudes to them
- » Physical availability to child and impairment of ability to provide care
- » Capacity to acknowledge risks to child
- » Emotional availability to child
- » Strategies to protect child from impact of mental health problems
- » Other risk factors and impact on parental relationship/partnership
- » Consistency and reliability
- » Previous parenting capacity

Bottom left box (Child's developmental needs):
- » Impact of behaviours brought about by parental mental health problems (or treatments) on basic care provided to child
- » Subsequent special health needs arising from the above and access (or barriers) to appropriate care and treatment
- » Effect on school attendance & ability to learn
- » Impact on quality of attachment(s) and feeling valued
- » Attitudes to treatments & professionals
- » Attitudes to seeking help
- » Capacity to seek help
- » Experience of loss/bereavement
- » Sibling relationships
- » Other caring relationships & 'lifelines'
- » Secrecy, stigma and social exclusion
- » Impact on friendships
- » Level of caring for self, parents & siblings
- » Impact of other significant risk factors such as parental substance misuse

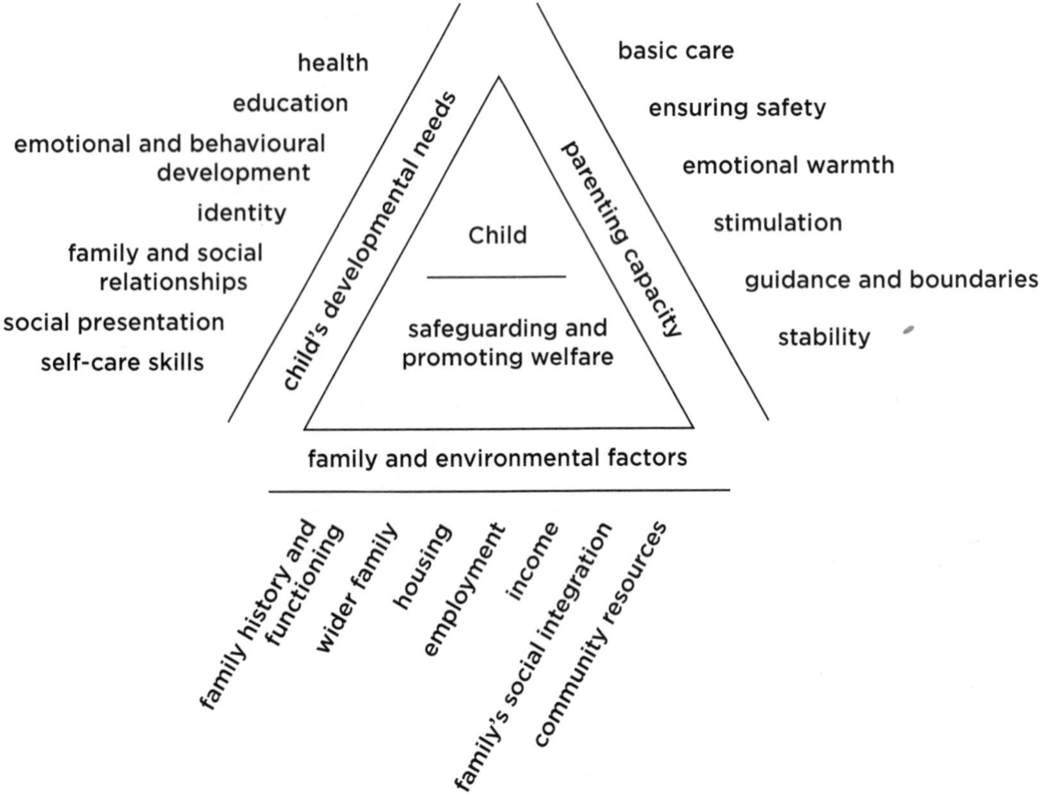

Bottom right box (Family and environmental factors):
- » Past treatment/engagement
- » Other risk factors in wider family
- » Who knows about problems and implications for wider family relationships
- » Extended family able to act as carers
- » Adequacy of material resources – money and housing
- » Level of community resources
- » Community attitudes and stigma
- » Support network outside the home

Working with coexisting/multiple needs

As already mentioned in Chapters 1 and 2, it is common for more than one parental difficulty (such as mental health problems and substance misuse) to coexist. Therefore, working effectively with families in these circumstances will involve understanding and addressing multiple needs. There is the added challenge of trying to 'unpick' the relationship between one difficulty and another. For example, this may mean exploring the questions: Is substance misuse a form of self-medication for a pre-existing mental health difficulty? Is a person's paranoia or depression caused or exacerbated by substance use? Where domestic abuse is present are alcohol or drugs a factor in increasing the likelihood of abusive incidents? Is a mental health difficulty such as depression caused by a person experiencing domestic abuse?

Understanding the above relationships is not easy and many people directly experiencing the situation may not know the answers to these questions themselves. However, it is worth seeking to understand the dynamics between one problem and another because doing so may lead to a more successful intervention and more targeted support. It can make it more possible to identify and deal with an underlying problem. It may also help to foresee and deal with challenges that can occur during a process of change. For example, if substance use is a way of coping or of numbing overwhelming feelings, the person trying to reduce their substance use may need help in finding an alternative way of managing these feelings.

Just as with all good assessments, the above involves 'hypothesising' (discussed earlier in this chapter on page 82). In the case of coexisting problems there is an added need to hypothesise about the interrelationship between one difficulty or behaviour and another. Furthermore, there is a need to hypothesise about the added impact of the combined issues on the child. How does the multiple nature of problems impact on risk, on harm and on how the child experiences and perceives things? Consciously hypothesising and seeking information to confirm or disconfirm these hypotheses will aid analysis, planning and intervention. However, that said, efforts to try and understand the relationship between factors should not be allowed to delay decision-making and taking timely actions needed to secure the welfare of a child (Galvani and Livingstone 2012).

Approaches to intervention

The needs and welfare of the child must remain firmly in focus throughout any work with children and families. Finely balanced judgements and decisions will have to be made. Work must be continuously and systematically reviewed to guard against the twin perils of *either* 'drift/distraction' on to the specific needs of adults *or* precipitating reactive practice. For the sake of the children involved, attempts to facilitate change should not be persisted in where parental resistance to it is such that it becomes clear families are unlikely or unwilling to change. In such circumstances, professionals must intervene to protect the child's welfare. The following are some considerations to help guide practice in an area where maintaining clarity and focus can be a challenge.

There can be a tendency for children's practitioners (from non-drug-specialist services) to push for total abstinence from parental drug use. This is not always necessary or realistic and an emphasis on total change can make it harder for parents to make smaller, more realistic changes. Initially, stabilising drug use and a harm-minimisation approach can be more realistic and helpful. Of course where service users desire abstinence, their efforts to achieve it should be supported, with awareness that the stress within the family may initially increase as a result. After all, substance use can be seen as a 'coping strategy' or, for some, as a form of 'self-medication', which will need replacing with alternative ways of coping.

An increased understanding of the nature of substance addiction and the process of change (or the Cycle of Change Model developed by Prochaska, Norcross and Diclemente (1994)) might help relevant professionals to better support such change. While the model is untested and has not been evaluated in work with children and families, in our view, it does have value as a framework which used skilfully and intelligently can help professionals to better understand how ready a person (particularly with an addiction or learned dependency) might be for change, help with engagement and with determining the nature, pace and timing of any support or interventions. It is important that the model is understood and not used in a simplistic manner. A key feature of the model is the acceptance that change is not easy and that people may need repeated opportunities to achieve the desired objective. Careful assessment of needs and risks and agreement of objectives are therefore critical. The nature of the intervention should be appropriate to the stage in the cycle at which the person seems to be. Additionally, harnessing the motivation of parents is key to the success of interventions.

Below we have made some adaptations to the model from Prochaska *et al.* (1994) further supplemented by adapted material from *Understanding the Change Process/Cycle of Change.*[3]

Cycle of change model[4]

1. Pre-contemplation
Parent sees no reason to change their behaviour – whatever the advice offered. The disadvantages of change outweigh advantages. Range of defence mechanisms are likely to be seen. Most commonly there's likely to be some degree of denial or minimisation of the problem. There could also be rationalisations (excuses such as 'I need drugs to relax') or projection/displacement (e.g. diagnosing own problem in someone else or locating problem on worker for removing child for example). Despite what might seem at first to be intractable difficulties there are some *strategies* that could work at this stage. These include:

---

3   See NRCFCPP Concurrent Permancy Planning Curriculum, Module 3: *Stages of Change.* Available at: www.hunter.cuny.edu/socwork/nrcfcpp/downloads/cpp/module3-stages_of_change.pdf.

4   Adaptation of text from pp.40–6: 'The Cycle of Change' from *Changing for Good* by James O. Prochaska, John C. Norcross and Carlo C. Diclemente. Copyright © 1994 by James O. Prochaska, John C. Norcross and Carlo C. Diclemente. Reprinted by permission of HarperCollins Publishers.

- providing information and feedback to raise problem awareness
- raising doubt to increase parent's perception of risks and problems with current behaviour
- helping them with a self-assessment
- identifying relationships that help
- creating awareness of defences especially in a therapeutic situation
- avoiding prescriptive advice, which is likely to be counterproductive and create further resistance to change.

2. Contemplation

The person considers making a change at some point in the future, but is still ambivalent and unsure about making a firm commitment to it. There's likely to be seesawing between consideration and rejection of change. *Strategies* at this stage include:

- eliciting reasons on both sides of the seesaw and tipping balance in favour of change
- double reflections help to clarify seesaw or ambivalent feelings
- using parent's language and goals.

3. Preparation for/decision to change

A decision to change is taken, and the person takes some personal responsibility for the desired changes and starts planning to take action. This presents a window of opportunity, open for a short time, for them either to advance or slip back. Suitable *strategies* include:

- articulating the choices in the parent's words
- suggesting choices
- probing their thoughts on the options
- goal setting
- identifying internal and external supports/resources
- identifying strategies to help change.

4. Action

The person actively pursues the desired change. Observable effort is made to break with old habits or to develop a new, more positive, one. *Strategies* likely to work include:

- cheering on
- supporting parent to take steps towards change
- reflecting back goals
- providing specific skill training/relevant programmes
- reviewing initial reasons that led to decision to change.

5. Maintenance

The desired change has been achieved and lasted for some time. The main task at this stage is to prevent oneself from slipping back into old habits (relapse prevention). Strategies include:

- helping to identify and use strategies to prevent relapse
- helping prepare for and expect relapse
- urging the person to continue on the wheel of change
- clarifying consequences
- not giving up.

Timing

Timing is very important in harnessing motivation, as delays can mean it is lost. Crisis theory and practice principles recognises a 'window of opportunity' that is presented in a crisis (when people's normal coping mechanisms break down) that is thought to last around four to six weeks (Roberts 1990, 2005). This provides potential opportunities for problem resolution and growth and for the integration of solutions-based therapies into the professional repertoire of responses. It is highly likely that referrals, whether from the family or from other agencies, will be made at a point of crisis for a child and/or parent and/or the wider family. Without proactive, helpful support and intervention during this window the likelihood of unhelpful or dysfunctional responses appearing or becoming fixed are increased. Service waiting times and complex processes can thus have a marked bearing on the outcomes for children and families.

Additionally, while it is important to consider each party's own needs in relation to timescales, there will be tensions because:

> the developing nature of a young child demands a different framework of time to the needs of a chronically ill parent or the bureaucratic needs of the court. (Gopfert *et al.* 2004, p.94)

This involves weighing up the developmental needs of a child against probable 'recovery' time for parents.

Strength and goal focus

Solution-focused, systemic interventions, in which it is assumed as a starting point that parents probably want the best for their children and will use services if offered appropriately, tend to be helpful. Studies report parents feeling that they are 'seen as a case' during assessments and of frustration at the emphasis on deficits and weaknesses. They often describe a stream of professionals continually focusing on weakness, which over time undermines their sense of their own abilities (Turnell and Edwards 1999). In *Signs of Safety: A Solution and Safety-orientated Approach to Child Protection*, Turnell and Edwards (1999) argue that there is only limited usefulness in assessments, which focus entirely on deficits (for example: Which needs aren't met? Which risks are present?). They argue that a greater focus on strengths and a better consideration of the goals and values of parents makes true partnership and collaboration far more likely. It is worth noting that taking a solutions-focused approach also works well with men. In their practice guide, the Fatherhood Institute and Family Rights Group suggest that professionals are more likely to be successful in sustaining engagement with fathers if they: 'adopt a strengths-based approach which supports the father's capabilities rather than treating him as an object of concern' (Fatherhood Institute 2012 p.11).

Questions framed to elicit strengths can generate useful information for families and professionals. If someone is unable to see any strengths or positives, this, in itself, could provide useful information.

In the *Signs of Safety* approach, Turnell and Edwards (1999) suggest the following ways of eliciting information about strengths.

- Use exception questions, such as 'Tell me about times when you/the parent has been managing well?' The question is based on assumptions that the problem isn't happening constantly and that the parent probably manages the problem some of the time. The answers elicited from questions such as this can uncover safe, constructive behaviours.

- Ensure that the detail of the 'exception' is explored, the *how, when, where and what*.

- Explore, knowing that it's possible, how confident the person is in their ability to repeat the exception.

Turnell and Edwards stress that this does involve a shift in conversation, so they recommend ensuring the 'problem' has been fully acknowledged before exploring exceptions, asking the question in three ways before moving on and not expecting people to be able to change their focus from the problem at the first time of asking.

Practitioners have commented to us about how much easier it is to bring up and engage in discussions about concerns and problems when an atmosphere of looking at positives has already been established. A strengths-based approach is not about just staying with what is comfortable, but also about there being more balance and engagement.

Another way of harnessing existing strengths and potential for change is through identifying the goals of service users. An explicit emphasis on goals is another feature of solution-focused approaches and the *Signs of Safety* model.

> Intake is a process of setting clear goal posts so that everybody knows what behaviour is expected and can clearly see when it has been achieved. (Hamer 2005, p.14)

If goals are coming primarily from professionals, it can be more helpful for them to focus on those elements which need to be present rather than on those which are currently absent, for example telling a parent they need to be in earshot and eyesight of the baby at all times rather than telling them to stop leaving the child unattended or unsupervised (Turnell and Edwards 1999). Also, when setting goals with (and ideally driven by) family members, these goals need to have clearly specified outcomes and be broken down into manageable steps. Achievable measures of success defined by parents are better than over-optimistic expectations. This helps to ensure that parents are not set up to fail. For example, in some cases substance use reduction or control is a more realistic goal than abstinence and can significantly increase family stability.

Within Brief Therapy[5] approaches, change is viewed as continuous, so one change will inevitably lead to another (Cade and O'Hanlon 1993). Focusing on specific small changes can lead to a sense of achievement, increased confidence and readiness for more, whereas big goals can be frustrating and undermine confidence.

Strengths and values cards (see practice example 4) are one approach to eliciting information from families about what things are important to them and what their values and goals are.

Practice example 4 shows how a family drug and alcohol service focuses on strengths and goals to encourage better outcomes for families.

Practice example 4: CASA Family Service, London

Since July 2006, CASA Family Service[6] has been offering an accessible therapeutic service to families affected by parental use of alcohol or other drugs. It helps families to build on their strengths and develop ways of minimising harm, caused by parental use of alcohol or other drugs, to family members and particularly to children and young people.

Background

CASA Family Service has grown out of the work of CASA, a voluntary-sector alcohol and drug service for adults based in North London. Over a number of years, CASA has developed services for parents and carers and was in a good position to develop a family service when the opportunity arose via commissioning from the local Drug and Alcohol Action Team (DAAT) in the London Borough of Islington.

This commissioning arrangement with the DAAT has positioned the service within an overall strategy of Hidden Harm services for children, young people and their families within the local borough of Islington – thus ensuring good multi-agency links across statutory and voluntary sector adults' and children's services from the outset.

---

5   Brief Therapy is an umbrella term for a variety of planned short-term, solution-oriented approaches. Approaches grew out of the work of therapists working at the Mental Research Institute, Palo Alto, CA in the 1970s.

6   For further information, contact: Chris Arnold, CASA Family Service Manager, 86 Durham Road, London N7 7DU, Tel: 020 7561 7490, Email: C.Arnold@blenheimcdp.org.uk

Practice approach

The work with families, and with the professional networks around them, aims to help parents and carers build up patterns of protective parenting and also increase the resilience of children and young people. After initial sessions with parents or carers on their own, parents and children are invited to attend weekly family sessions together, during which a semi-structured model of intervention is followed. The model was developed by Wendy Robinson as a practice approach called Child-Focused Family Intervention.

Family values and strengths cards

An integral part of this approach is the use of card-sort exercises to start therapeutic conversations with families in the first few sessions. These are engaging and accessible to children of all ages, as well as to adults, and offer families the space to talk more readily about their family circumstances and personal views. The card-sort exercises are particularly designed to invite families to talk about: what matters most to them in their family life; which of these things get affected by difficulties such as parental use of alcohol or drugs; and what strengths and resources they have to build on. Often families find that this process allows them to identify more clearly how they want family life to be and how it currently is, or has been, affected by parental use of alcohol or drugs. This process can lead to a strong sense of motivation to change while also encouraging a family's sense of confidence to achieve manageable change. Within this strengths-based approach, CASA particularly works with families to identify parenting strengths in order to create a safer and more secure family environment.

- Following the card-sort exercises, families are enabled to identify manageable goals for change in their work with the service – primarily in relation to alcohol or other drug use, parenting and children's needs. These goals are shared with referrers where appropriate and are reviewed with the family at regular intervals. In addition to family sessions, there is direct work with children or parents and carers on an individual basis; interventions are tailored to the particular needs and choices of each family.

Collaborative working with support networks

CASA has found it helpful to take a proactive and collaborative stance with families and the professional networks with which they often engage. In order to work with the whole system of support around family members, CASA aims to find a balance between prioritising client confidentiality within its therapeutic work with making clear agreements about sharing information with other professionals when this is supportive to family members.

Working with resistance

Forms of resistance – such as denial and minimisation of problems – are often associated with addiction but also apply to other problems that people find too difficult to face or that make them feel immobilised. Working with resistance is very challenging and many professionals have little training or preparation in responding to this constructively.

Approaches that involve challenging and confronting people or 'trying to make them see or admit' to the extent of their problems, tend to increase the likelihood of people feeling defensive or feeling the need to hide things even more and of them withdrawing. This poses considerable challenges for practitioners in statutory children and families services who often use such approaches when there are child protection concerns. Practitioners in such services, and in fact all practitioners trying to engage with people who they feel are resistant, should consider critically the extent to which their practices are unintentionally reinforcing such denial.

Miller and Rollnick (2002) argue that good empathic listening, which is at the heart of their Motivational Interviewing approach, is far more productive. They describe it as 'a collaborative conversational style for strengthening a person's own motivation and commitment to change'(Miller and Rollnick 2012).

There is strong evidence that Motivational Interviewing (MI) works in brief interventions (Treasure 2004, and see also the Royal College of Psychiatrists website[7]). In many controlled trials, the approach has been found to be almost always effective; it has been effective in relation to alcohol and substance misuse, medication compliance, dual diagnosis, mental illness treatment and eating disorders.

The principles of the approach are broadly compatible with core social work values. It is client centred and empathic, considers ambivalence to be a normal and ordinary part of the change process, involves collaborating with service users and guides them towards change. It does this through:

- understanding
- giving choice and control
- questioning in a curious, open, empathic way and using 'change talk'.

Miller and Rollnick set out the following components of the approach and some general principles (Miller and Rollnick 2002, p.34).

---

7   www.rcpsych.ac.uk

The Motivational Interviewing (MI) approach[8]

There are three key components of the MI approach: collaboration, evocation and autonomy.

- **Collaboration** – involves counsellor and client working together towards goals that emerge from their collaboration. It requires the counsellor/interviewer to be aware of the attitudes and goals that they themselves bring to the interpersonal relationship. It also involves the creation of a positive atmosphere 'conducive to change'.

- **Evocation** – involves 'drawing out' (like water from a well) the intrinsic motivation from the person, not 'imparting'.

- **Autonomy** – refers to the fact that the responsibility for change must lie with the client. When MI is done properly, it's the client not the counsellor who presents the arguments for change.

- **Express empathy** – as it is fundamental to effectiveness (as described by Rogers 1962) and the 'acceptance' of people 'as they are' is crucial and seems to free people up to change. Conversely, family therapists use a term – 'ironic process' – where an action causes the response it is designed to prevent, for example saying 'you have to change' immobilises people. Ambivalence is accepted as a normal part of human experience and not pathology.

- **Develop discrepancy** – as MI can be intentionally directive (unlike person-centred counselling). The goal is to amplify the discrepancy between the person's behaviour and their goals or values.

- **Roll with resistance** – otherwise, if the counsellor advocates change and the client argues against it, it is counterproductive and may even push the client further in the opposite direction. In MI, the counsellor doesn't 'oppose resistance, but rolls or flows with it' and resistance is a signal to shift approach. New perspectives are invited (from the client by turning questions or problems back on the person) and not imposed.

---

8   Miller, W. R. and Rollnick, S. (2002) *Motivational Interviewing: Preparing People for Change.* New York: Guilford Press. Used with permission of Guilford Press.

- **Support self-efficacy** – as this term refers to a person's belief in his or her ability to succeed with something and is an important part of motivation. A counsellor's belief in a client's ability to change can create a self-fulfilling prophecy. The authors raise some concerns with the notion of 'resistance', which implies one person is resistant (they think it is more relational than that). In the latest edition, the authors have chosen to replace this with the concept of 'discord'. In their view 'the phenomenon of discord signals dissonance in your working alliance' (Miller and Rolnick 2012, p.211).

Forrester argues that social workers (and others) would benefit from applying the principles of an MI approach in their work. Through research, Forrester found that for some practitioners, basic training in the approach improved listening skills and resulted in a less-confrontational style, a reduced tendency to impose a social work agenda and, as a result, an increased ability to engage constructively with service users (Forrester 2004; Forrester *et al.* 2008).

The term 'Motivational Interviewing' strictly applies to the use of the approach by fully trained clinicians, and Miller and Rollnick (2012) are clear that it is not a 'technique', preferring to describe it as 'a style of being with people, an integration of particular clinical skills to foster motivation for change' (p.35). However, other practitioners can draw on some of the methods, and most importantly the underlying principles, and this can benefit their approach. Substance-misuse professionals are commonly trained in the approach. Because of its noted success for working with ambivalence and resistance, there is a growing interest in MI training for wider groups of professionals, with some areas making it a key plank in their staff training and development strategy.

Direct support to children

When asked what has helped them, children tend to refer to help from family members, informal mentors and friends rather than the actions of paid professionals. Although most children prefer to talk to peers of their own age, knowing there is an adult with a listening ear at the right time can prove crucial.

An awareness of the potential helpfulness of sources of informal support is vital if professionals are to ensure that their intervention does not weaken these links.

Considering how support can strengthen and build on resilience factors for children (outlined in Chapter 3) is an important starting point when considering appropriate support for children.

Many children compartmentalise aspects of their lives in order to cope with situation and many experience feelings of guilt and a sense of responsibility for parents' problems. They need help, encouragement and sometimes skilled interver...on to enable them to share their feelings.

When asked about their experiences of stress, whereas adults tend to point to major stressful life events, children and young people refer to 'daily hassles' (Newman and Blackburn 2002, p.6), such as falling out with friends. Such events and stresses should not be overlooked given their capacity to cause feelings of stress in children, because cumulative or chronic stress presents potentially long-term risks to children and young people.

In her review of the research and literature relating to parental mental ill health, Tunnard (2004) listed the following responses of children as to what they wanted in terms of support.

They wanted:

- above all for their parent or parents to be well
- for themselves to be cared for
- to get the attention they need
- for their parents to be able to meet other parents in similar circumstances
- information – children and young people want to understand:
  - the reason for their parent's mood swings
  - medication
  - the causes of mental illness
  - symptoms
  - likely consequences of health problems
  - how to deal with problems
  - when to call a GP
  - how to notice changes in mood and their significance
- help in coping with embarrassing or bizarre behaviours that their parent exhibits in public, in school or in front of their peers
- information to be age-appropriate and not overloading
- someone to talk to
- opportunities to relax and have fun.

(Adapted from Tunnard 2002a)

According to Tunnard (2002a), children affected by parental substance misuse have many similar wishes and often need:

- time away
- reassurance that their parent's drug use is not their fault or responsibility
- help with losses and separations

- help and reassurance concerning fears of being removed from their home or parent (real or imagined)
- opportunities for group discussion and activities (these may be inclusive as opposed to specialist, as this is often better received and has benefits)
- the above to be in tandem with changes at home (perhaps brought about by a parent benefiting from treatment)
- either individual or family work to help the child to find ways of coping with changes, new rules and boundaries
- respite and recreation opportunities.

(Adapted from Tunnard 2002a)

In direct work, going at a pace appropriate to children's needs and circumstances is not an easy balance to strike and requires skill and awareness of the child's communication needs and level of development.

As with adults, identifying children's goals, strengths, likes and dislikes provides a useful foundation for working with them. Engaging them in activities they enjoy often results in them communicating a lot more freely than when using more formal approaches. Practitioners can use a range of creative and engaging tools and techniques such as trigger cards, manuals, workbooks, social stories, ecomaps and variations thereof, sand play and games in their direct work with children. Communicating by email and text has also increased the likelihood of children and young people keeping in touch with services.

Practice example 5 describes a holistic service for families affected by parental substance misuse, which gives support to help parents and children play together. Within the service is also provision for young people using drugs or alcohol or concerned about a family member, friend or carer who is.

Practice example 5: CAN, Northamptonshire

CAN[9] offers a holistic service to families where parents recognise that their substance use is impacting on the care of their children. As well as undertaking individual counselling, group work and advice and support with adults, CAN Children's Workers work on a one-to-one basis with service users' children aged 5–12. The Children's Workers use lots of tactile resources to help with the communication of feelings through play. This includes the use of sand trays, puppets, board games, books, dolls and figures, paints, Play-Doh, etc. The parent(s)/carer(s) are involved in the work with the children from the start. They are invited to attend an appointment in order that the Children's Worker can complete an assessment for the child/ren. They are then invited to attend review sessions with the worker every six weeks to discuss the work that has been completed with the child/ren and to help them communicate in an

---

9   For further information about CAN, contact: Ellie Davies and Sue Becker at CAN Northampton, Tel: 01604 627027 Anthea Spence (Children's Worker), Tel: 01933 271879 or 01604 627027

age-appropriate way with their child about their substance use issues and its impact on the child. It was partly during these sessions that it was identified that some service users find it difficult to play with their children. This could be for a variety of reasons. It might be that the client did not experience play with their own parent(s) or that their misuse is their primary concern and play is not high on the agenda. In response to this need, CAN staff organise Play Workshops throughout the year and with individual families working with the service, which have proved very successful. Clients with children are invited to come along and do various activities together. The team are on hand to join in as well as answer any questions the parent(s)/carer(s) might have.

CAN Young People's Team service

CAN Young People's Team (CAN YP Team) is a free, confidential drug and alcohol service for young people under the age of 19 and their families/carers in Northamptonshire. CAN YP Team aims to provide information, education, advice and treatment to young people in relation to drug and alcohol use.[10]

Who can access CAN YP Team?

- A young person who is concerned about someone else's drug use including parents, carers, siblings or friends.
- A young person who is using but would like to reduce the harm caused.
- A young person who would like to reduce their drug use or stop.
- A young person who needs an opiate substitute prescription (methadone, Subutex).
- A young person who needs support into inpatient detox for alcohol dependency.

What is on offer?

- Confidential information, education and harm-reduction advice around drug and alcohol use.
- Referral into treatment.
- BBV (Blood Borne Viruses) screening.
- Family work.
- Relapse work and aftercare.

---

10 For further information, contact: Admin base at 76 St Giles Street, Northampton NN1 1JW, Tel: 08450 556246, Email: ypadmin@can.org.uk, Fax: 01604 930035

- Group information, education and harm-reduction sessions for targeted groups.
- Work with looked-after children.
- Dedicated Schools Liaison Worker.
- Exploitation prevention and awareness work.
- Joint work with the youth offending service and the police.
- Advice for professionals.
- Professionals' training sessions.

Practice example 6 concerns a service with a focus on early intervention. In this instance a project for Asian teenage girls has enhanced accessibility to service users and engaged their parents, community leaders and other professionals.

Practice example 6: Newham Asian Women's Project

Zindaagi (meaning 'life') is a project led by Newham Asian Women's Project (NAWP).[11] The project delivers a range of services aimed at reducing the incidence of self-harm and suicide amongst South Asian women and girls and actively works to promote their emotional well-being and self-empowerment.

Its early intervention project involves workshops and drop-in sessions in schools as well as after-school clubs, Teens@NAWP and Girls Allowed, for young women. Workshops are delivered on a range of issues, such as confidence building, self-esteem, stress management, etc. To increase accessibility, the team has adapted the way it works and after sessions drop the girls back home. Parents feel more comfortable seeing the children being dropped off and knowing who they are with. As a result, the project has built a trusting relationship with parents who then allow their daughters to go on residential weekend trips with the group as well.

Providing workshops and the service in schools has proved to be very successful, especially given that many South Asian parents do not want their children to be out after school. Having a presence in school provides them with the opportunity to access services they may not otherwise be able to, as well as ensuring that it is a setting in which they are comfortable.

In order to communicate more effectively with young women, the team has also begun to use an office mobile phone. This allows the young women to text or leave a missed call if they need to talk. This is a medium of communication they are comfortable using and means that they can be texted with reminders of meetings, etc. This is a method that is age-appropriate and has enabled larger numbers of young women to access the services.

---

11   For further information, contact: Zindaagi Team, Newham Asian Women's Project 661, Barking Road, Plaistow London E13 9EX, Tel: 0208 472 0528, 079 6164 4088, Email: info@nawp.org

The services are user led and developed. The team consistently consults with service users on their needs and how they would like the service to develop. Creative methods of evaluation have involved getting the young women to keep a diary of how they felt before and after activities, what's worked for them and what hasn't, and this also allows the team to gauge their emotional growth.

In addition, to increase professionals' awareness of the cultural issues impacting on young women and the effect these may have on the way they engage with mental health services, the service delivers training to professionals highlighting some of these cultural concepts.

The team also works within the community with faith leaders who are often the first point of contact for many BAMER (Black and Minority Ethnic or Refugee) young women experiencing emotional distress. Providing them with the knowledge and information to support their clients appropriately is important and also helps to dispel some of the myths that are held by the community at large about mental health.

Quotes from people who have used or worked with the Zindaagi project

I used to get bullied and the bullying workshop has helped me learn how to deal with bullies…I feel happier that now I know I can do something about it…I feel that I would be able to talk to Teens [youth group] or to my parents if it happens again. (Young Asian woman)

I felt it was a very safe and warm environment that generated in-depth discussions. The trainers were knowledgeable and made us very comfortable from the start. Raised my awareness of self-harm and issues of the Asian communities. (Professional's evaluation of self-harm training, and young Asian women)

Support to parents

Research and literature consistently shows that when asked what they wanted, the majority of parents with mental health problems referred first to what they wanted for their children: to feel ordinary and to get early attention and support if their life is disrupted (Tunnard 2004). When asked about what would help them in terms of support, although there are some differences, there is much commonality between what those affected by parental substance misuse and mental health issues have said. Parents often report feeling undermined. They do not want to be judged or in fear of their children being removed if they ask for help. They require professionals to be proactive in giving reassurance about negative perceptions they think they may hold about them, as they are used to stigmatising and discriminating attitudes (Tunnard 2004). While this section uses the term 'parent' throughout, much will apply to alternative carers or other affected family members. If/when relevant, specific considerations pertaining to fathers are highlighted.

Help in their own right

Many parents, particularly those with mental health problems, say they want help to meet their parental responsibilities. Parents whose children undertake caring roles generally want support to relieve the burden on the child (a few parents with severe mental health problems were not troubled by children caring for them, but most didn't want to be so reliant on their children) (Tunnard 2004).

Since the publication of the first edition of this handbook, there has been a noticeable growth in bids to replicate or to adapt and evaluate evidence-based programmes (practice example 7 falls into this category).

Practice example 7 describes an intensive parenting programme that has been developed to work specifically with substance-misusing parents of newborn babies and aims to help them to achieve their parenting goals.

Practice example 7: Parents Under Pressure

Parents Under Pressure (PUP) is an intensive parenting programme that was originally developed in Australia.[12] Working with methadone-dependent mothers with children aged two to eight years, the PUP programme was shown as part of a randomised control trial (RCT) trial to achieve a reduction in child abuse potential, parenting stress and child behaviour problems.

UK study

The NSPCC is working with the programme developers to test the effectiveness of the PUP programme in 11 centres across the UK.[13] The programme has been developed to work specifically with substance misusing parents of newborn babies and infants aged up to two-and-a-half years. An independent RCT and a wider service evaluation are currently being undertaken by the University of Warwick in order to measure the impacts of the programme and its cost effectiveness and fit with UK delivery systems. Specific outcome measures for the UK trial include evidence of an improvement in parent–infant interaction, reduction in child abuse and potential for child abuse, improved parenting and reduction in family stress. The evaluation will also address rates of substance misuse and capacity to sustain change through a six-month follow-up period. The NSPCC PUP service is working with parents who misuse alcohol as well as those who misuse illegal drugs.

---

12 www.pupprogram.net.au

13 For further information, contact: Gwynne Rayns NSPCC Development Manager, Email: grayns@ nspcc.org.uk

This is one of the first large-scale European studies to examine a programme targeting the parenting of substance-dependent parents of infants in terms of its effectiveness in improving the parent–infant relationship and reducing the potential for child maltreatment. The findings of the RCT study will be available in December 2016.

Practice model

The programme is a manualised, home-based intervention that is underpinned by an ecological model of child development and targets multiple dimensions of family functioning. It addresses the psychological functioning of individuals in the family, the parent–child relationship and social–contextual factors such as social isolation, accommodation and financial issues. The key mechanisms for achieving change in families are the ecological approach, the therapeutic alliance with parents and a focus on mindfulness to help improve parental affect regulation.

The programme is delivered on a one-to-one basis within the family home. Parents receive a Parent Workbook, which forms the basis of the programme and contains many different exercises that help parents work towards their parenting goals. Comprising 12 modules, the PUP practitioner uses the programme creatively, tailoring the use of the modules to reflect the unique needs and resources of each family.

Each PUP practitioner has to work with three families and complete a written case study in order to achieve accreditation. To support their development, practitioners receive three days' training in the model and additional clinical supervision.

Case study

Millie and Nathan's story

I was referred to the PUP programme because social services were worried that I wasn't giving my two-year-old son, Nathan, enough attention to meet his needs. I had suffered from domestic violence when I was younger and I was drinking a lot to black out my problems. I would get drunk so that I didn't have to deal with the pain or with the stresses of my current relationships. A few years earlier I'd mixed myself a big cocktail of different drinks and then tried to cut my wrists and I was heading that way again.

I'd drink two or three times a week and once I started I didn't know when to stop. I didn't think about the effect on my children. When I was hung-over, I didn't have the energy to play with them. I wasn't there for them when they wanted to speak to me and I often scared them by snapping at them. I would see to Nathan's physical needs by feeding him and changing him, but I didn't have the energy to cuddle or play with him, a lot of the time I ignored him as I was so wrapped up in my own problems. I had low confidence and low self-esteem and I would cry all the time. I didn't value myself or even like myself. I didn't leave the house other than to take the older two to school and to go to case conferences to decide the future of the children.

During the PUP programme I realised I was scaring the kids by screaming at them and sometimes I was timid and wouldn't stand up for myself. I learnt that I could play with my children but that I also needed to be more assertive. I was taught to cope with my panic attacks and how to calm myself down when I felt one coming on. This was a big turning point for me. The panic attacks were brought on by the stress in my life and I realised that I'd used alcohol to block out some problems from my past and once I stopped drinking I had to face things.

If it wasn't for the PUP programme my kids would still have been on the Child Protection Plan. My relationship with my children has improved no end and I'm a lot more loving with them. I'm a lot happier now and so are they. When I was drinking all the time I didn't realise things could even be as good as they are now.

Practical and emotional support

Whilst some parents want parenting advice, research by the ESRC Families and Social Capital Research Group at South Bank University (Edwards and Gillies 2005) shows that most would prefer concrete, practical services. Services that 'lighten the load' or alleviate stress, such as help with transporting children to school, are valued (Tunnard 2004). Also, parents appreciate being able to gain support from other parents and being enabled to have a break. Substance-misusing parents particularly value access to informal support during difficult times and help with practical and emotional problems that might not be substance related (Kroll and Taylor 2003). Childcare support being available when needed and services that help to reduce isolation are also wanted, and there is a greater need for follow up and aftercare services than is generally currently available.

Emotional support that parents indicate would be helpful includes:

- help in coping with children's needs when they have emotional and behavioural difficulties
- support to help family members understand each other
- counselling or someone to talk to informally or both
- assistance in finding alternative coping styles, if they are needing to change, or in reducing the use of their usual strategies.

A practical support need often cited by parents is for accessible, clear information. Parents would like to be given accessible information regarding the context of statutory services' role when they are involved with them, such as information about procedures, confidentiality and professionals' powers (Tunnard 2004). An additional consideration for fathers is the need to spell out their specific role in plans so that they do not assume 'parent' means 'mother' (*Community Care* 2012). Information about medication and its effects, and for substance-misusing parents, information sensitively provided about the impact of parents' substance use on their children, is also wanted (Morris and Wates 2006).

Preventative support and help in promoting resilience

Professional involvement at an early stage is wanted by many parents and not just during a crisis. Heidi Lloyd, a mother who had experienced mental health difficulties described in Falkov (1998) draws on her own experience of parenting with mental health problems and suggests that parents can benefit from doing things to help reduce stress, for example by having enough food in to cover meals for at least two days in case they become tired or unwell, having a few convenience meals to hand, preparing lunchboxes and clothes for the children for the next day in advance. Such strategies, if individually developed and tailored, can help people to feel in control and 'stop the day seeming so overwhelming'.

Practice example 8 provides a case study to illustrate how one service worked with a family at an early stage. This example looks at the service to one family. Further information on the service more generally is covered in practice example 9.

Practice example 8: Family Action case study from a London Building Bridges service

Building Bridges is a home-based family support service that works with families with multiple complex needs in order to make families stronger, safer and more fulfilling for children and parents.[14]

Case study

Anita is married with a two-year-old daughter and was referred to a Family Action Building Bridges service in London. She had previously been admitted to hospital once for her psychotic condition and had become overweight, anxious and mainly housebound, relying on her husband to care for her and their daughter. Both Anita and her husband were unemployed and had got into debt. Whenever Anita's mental health improved, her husband seemed to sabotage her progress. One serious incident involved Anita being filmed having a psychotic episode and her husband pushing their daughter to Anita, obviously distressing the child. Their daughter was beginning to display language development and behavioural problems, which was an additional stress for Anita.

The Building Bridges service worked with Anita, her husband and their daughter to understand the whole family's needs. The support worker helped

14 For further information, contact: Jayne Stokes, Email: jayne.stokes@family-action.org.uk or visit: www.family-action.org.uk

Anita to develop an insight into her mental health condition and establish a routine based on earlier waking and bedtimes, healthier eating and more exercise. These factors are known to support medication and impact positively on mental health in their own right. The worker accompanied Anita on shopping trips and to a local leisure centre to give her confidence in leaving the house. She showed Anita the importance of engaging with her daughter and how she could play with her in more creative ways. She also demonstrated to Anita and her husband how their inconsistent parenting approaches were causing some of their daughter's behavioural problems and engaged Anita's husband in understanding how he could be undermining Anita as a parent.

Since being helped by the Building Bridges service Anita and her daughter are exhibiting much-improved parent–child attachment. Her daughter's speech, behaviour and self-esteem have improved considerably and she has been found a nursery place close to home. Anita got a job but the stress involved in the change threatened relapse. She wants to try again in the future. In the meantime, Anita is studying childcare and volunteering for a mental health charity locally, has made some friends at the leisure centre with whom she is going swimming regularly and has lost more than a stone in weight. Her husband is taking driving lessons, volunteers in a community centre and has stopped smoking. The couple have reviewed their household budget to reduce their debt and have obtained permanent housing in better condition.

Learning points

- To secure improvements in outcomes for the child, the needs of the whole family should be approached holistically.

- As is shown by research into what works in family support, the role of a key worker who works consistently in partnership with the family is crucial.

- An all-important foundation for securing improvement in the child's outcomes is the creation of routines and structures to assist the parent with managing their difficulties.

- Other adults in a household may not have a presenting problem, but their behaviours may be impacting negatively on parent–child relationships and the child's behaviour and development. They may need support to understand why.

- Support needs to be given to parents not only with their relationships within the home but also with wider communities so that parents can begin to generate their own social networks. This can then provide ongoing support.

Flexible and holistic support services

Support services that are flexible and responsive to individual need, do not impose expectations and recognise the environmental factors that affect people are valued by families. Those that make proactive efforts to ensure provision is acceptable and inclusive of fathers are better able to engage and support them. For all parents, the opportunity to choose from a range of support services promotes their usefulness and uptake.

Voluntary services can often be tailored to family circumstances and play a very important role in supporting parents.

If parents can get their needs and those of the child met in the same place, the child is more likely to be seen and their needs addressed. Also, if parents can get a range of issues addressed in one place they are more likely to attend the service. 'One-stop shops' have been mentioned many times as a useful means of service provision.

Engaging with and using services can be time consuming and potentially stressful, particularly if childcare needs or other access issues are not addressed by the service. Services that are able to offer flexible appointment times, a choice of home visits or office/centre visits and drop-in facilities are more likely to be used.

Drawing specialists into convenient or comfortable (for service users) settings, such as trusted local voluntary or community services, can minimise the stress and anxiety that can come with having lots of appointments with different people and in different places.

Some specific service deficits, cited in surveys and studies as requiring improvements in order to better meet parents' support needs, include better family-friendly facilities in psychiatric hospitals, mother and baby units for women experiencing postnatal psychosis and support with bonding when babies in special care units have withdrawal symptoms (Morris and Wates 2006).

Supporting the whole family

For this we can look to ecological approaches, i.e. those that invite us to focus more widely on child, parent, family, wider networks and community.

> Ecological approaches rest on the premise that development and behaviour of individuals can be fully understood only in the context of the environments in which they live. Ecological theories, unlike other behavioural and psychological theories have a focus on systems and in particular on the interrelational transactions between systems. In the context of working with children and families this entails the use of a systems framework to examine relationships and mutual influences between child, family, friends, neighbours, communities, wider society. It is a holistic perspective which focuses on the ways in which children's developmental needs, the capacity of their parents to respond appropriately to those needs and wider environmental factors interact with one another over time. (NSPCC 2000, p.41)

The logical and perhaps unsurprising conclusion from this approach would be that interventions that are based on a clear and full assessment of the social support available and that increase supportive potential and decrease the stressful content are likely to be most effective.

Whole-family focus

Much has been said already about the need for professionals, both individually and collectively, to widen their thinking – particularly if they are from a service that is primarily set up for individual family members – to include the families of which those members are a part.

By widening thinking or 'thinking family' (Gopfert *et al.* 2004; SCIE 2011), it is possible to better understand individual members in terms of the pressures on them, the role they play and the knock-on effects of their feelings or behaviour on others and vice versa. As previously discussed, it is particularly important that fathers/'hidden men' are given due consideration.

It can be helpful to explore with individual service users (or all family members) what a typical day is like for them. By thinking about what happens for one person in this kind of detail, it can make it easier to imagine how others who live with them experience this. Gaining a clearer understanding of these factors will enable services to better support families, identify where gaps and needs are and target helpful interventions.

There are now a growing number of good or promising practice and service examples taking a whole-family focus, including some with a strong and growing evidence base. A number of these are outlined below.

Practice example 9 shows a parental mental health service operating a 'whole-family' approach.

Practice example 9: Family Action's Building Bridges project

Building Bridges is Family Action's home-based family support service that works with families with multiple complex needs in order to make families stronger, safer and more fulfilling for children and parents. The service has been running since 1999 and is currently delivered in Lewisham, Southwark, Newham, Tower Hamlets and Greenwich.[15]

Building Bridges works with families that might have problems such as parental mental illness, a young carer at home, difficulties in parenting, children with mental health or behavioural difficulties, relationship issues, safeguarding issues and financial and material hardship.

The service specification and arrangements for referrals to the service depend on local commissioning. However, the starting point for the service is families' perceptions of their needs and their goals. The service is delivered by professional Family Support Workers who provide practical as well as emotional support and are available at times when other services are not, such as at bedtimes, weekends and bank holidays.

---

15 For further information, contact: Jayne Stokes, Email: jayne.stokes@family-action.org.uk or visit: www.family-action.org.uk

Family Action works holistically in the family home with parents and children to develop an action plan that will help families build stronger and more positive futures. The service works with families to:

- promote good health
- meet emotional needs
- keep children safe
- feel part of their community
- support learning
- set boundaries
- encourage work aspirations
- provide a stable home
- manage their finances
- manage routines.

For example, where the service is commissioned by Tower Hamlets Council the focus is on supporting parents with mental health problems to manage their health better, reducing the need for higher-tier services and helping their children to feel safer at home. The service also works to improve children's understanding of their parent's health problems and improve family relationships, leading to better behavioural outcomes and school achievement.

Through the 'Family Star™ the service monitors each family's progress in the areas listed previously. The Family Star enables the service to track families' achievements and identify areas where extra support may be needed.

Figure 5.5: Example Family Star™

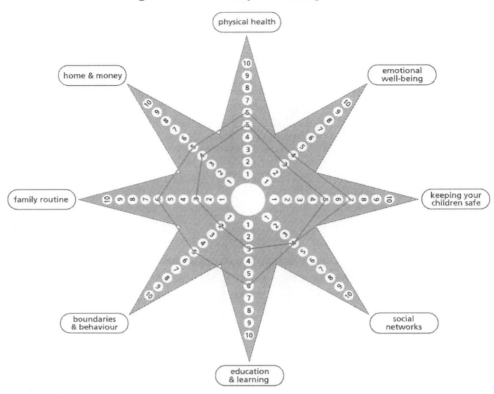

Family Star™ (2nd edition) © Triangle Consulting Social Enterprise Ltd Authors: Sarah Burns and Joy Mackeith www.outcomesstar.org

A C4EO (Centre for Excellence and Outcomes in Children and Young People) analysis of Building Bridges which features in their *Grasping the Nettle* report showed that: 'Over the course of one year, 40 families can be supported by Family Action's Building Bridges service at a cost of £3,500 per family. Over two years, the estimated savings to: the Department for Education and local authority are £114,400; the Department for Work and Pensions are £158,400; and the NHS are £67,200.'

An independent evaluation in 2011 found that the Building Bridges service resulted in a:

- 53 per cent reduction in needing a Care Programme Approach
- 46 per cent reduction in child protection plans
- 30 per cent reduction in children entering local authority care

- 48 per cent reduction in providing a common assessment framework team around the child – single agency

- 33 per cent reduction in providing a common assessment team around the child – multi-agency

- 46 per cent reduction in Children in Need (as per Section 17 Children Act 1989).

Practice example 10 shows how coordinated support for both a mother and her child can enhance their relationship and improve their circumstances. It illustrates family-focused direct work in action.

Practice example 10: ADAS UK

Synopsis of family situation

At the time of referral to the Child Therapy service at ADAS, Jack* was eight. His mother, Sarah,* contacted ADAS,[16] as she had concerns about his behaviour, describing him as withdrawing from her and trying to self-harm. Sarah had a history of drug use and alcohol misuse, although at the time of referral, she was no longer using drugs but was still binge drinking. Jack's father, Dean,* also had a history of drug use and, at the time of referral, was reported to be still using. Sarah and Dean no longer lived together and there was a history of domestic violence between them.

Sarah and Jack had recently spent time in a refuge and Jack had intermittent contact with his father.

The child therapist set up an initial referral meeting with Sarah. The aim of this meeting was to explore with Sarah what her concerns were regarding her son and also to obtain a fuller history of the family's main experiences. During this first meeting, Sarah talked about her long history of physical and mental ill health, her substance misuse difficulties and her recognition of the impact that all this had had on Jack, both when he was a baby and in recent years. Sarah admitted that Jack had taken on a great deal of responsibility, especially in looking after her. Sarah explained that Jack frequently missed school when she was too ill to leave the home and would take on household tasks such as cleaning and preparing simple meals for both of them. Sarah explained that for a while she had had a support worker from the refuge that she and Jack lived in but since being rehoused that support had ceased. Sarah and Jack were fairly isolated as a family unit in the new community they were living in. Following years of chaotic family life, Sarah had become estranged from most of her family and Jack had little contact with his father's family. Although Sarah was no longer using drugs, she was finding it increasingly difficult to cope with daily life stressors and

---

16 For further information, contact:Gareth Clement, Chief Executive, ADAS, 118–124 The Stow, Harlow, Essex, CM20 3AS, Tel: 01279 641347, Email: gareth.clement@adasuk.org or visit: www.adasuk.org

was concerned about the risk of starting to use again. She was also worried about her binge drinking, as she felt her alcohol intake was increasing.

During this first meeting and in a second follow-up meeting, the child therapist discussed the option of individual counselling for Sarah, some relapse prevention sessions and the possibility of Sarah working with a family support worker at ADAS. The child therapist also discussed what protective factors, if any, were in place when Sarah and Jack were alone at home. The child therapist also talked to Sarah about undertaking a Common Assessment Framework (CAF) with her and Jack, as it was deemed that Jack was a 'child in need'. Sarah said that Jack's school had already completed something similar and the child therapist sought consent from Sarah to contact Jack's school and find out if anything was already in place. Sarah agreed to these suggestions. It was also agreed that Sarah would start her own counselling before play therapy commenced with Jack to ensure that Sarah was able to contain Jack emotionally and to support him through his therapeutic intervention. The child therapist agreed to meet with Sarah on a regular basis to help her think of ways to facilitate communication between Sarah and Jack.

Action

Counselling for Sarah started shortly after the initial meetings with the Child Therapy service, and Jack's own play therapy sessions started a few weeks after that. In addition to that support, following an assessment by a support worker at ADAS, Sarah was found to be alcohol dependent and was referred to the local Community Drug and Alcohol Team (CDAT) where she was prescribed Antabuse to help her reduce her alcohol intake.

When a family is seen at ADAS by both the Adult and Child and Family services, regular family meetings are held, which are attended by the counsellor/s, child therapist and family support workers who are involved with the adult/s and child/ren. Confidentiality is maintained for both the adult/s and child/ren during these meetings but any issues that seem to be presenting difficulties for the family as a unit are discussed and any child protection concerns are highlighted and duly addressed; practical issues are also raised such as housing or financial issues. If these are seen to be causing further stress for the parent and/or child, the ADAS support worker is asked to work with the family. Communication between mother and son was raised by both the adult counsellor and the child therapist as being a difficulty and this was addressed with Sarah and Jack in a variety of ways. The Child Therapy service offers regular review meetings to parents in which themes and issues arising from the child's sessions are discussed. These were held with Sarah but in addition, she was also offered the opportunity to attend parenting support meetings with the family worker at ADAS where parenting strategies were discussed. Sarah attended these meetings regularly.

During the course of Sarah and Jack's engagement with ADAS, substantial progress was made by both mother and child. By having a safe space in which to express and explore his thoughts and feelings through the medium of play, Jack was able to move from being a withdrawn, highly anxious child to one whose self-esteem developed and who became able to express himself verbally. His relationship with his mother improved as her own self-esteem and confidence grew. Sarah did not revert to using drugs and was able to address her drinking difficulties through her counselling and the support from CDAT. The family worker was instrumental in helping Sarah regain her role as mother and this then allowed Jack to give up his 'parent' role that he had adopted. Sarah also learnt to listen to her son and to spend positive time with him. Although attempts were made by the Child and Family service at ADAS to engage with Jack's father, these were never successful and Jack's relationship with Dean continued to be difficult for him. Sarah was supported in trying to establish consistent contact between Jack and Dean but by the time this family left ADAS after just over a year of attending, contact between father and son continued to be problematic.

The relative success of the above intervention with Sarah and Jack was due to close collaboration between the Adult and Child and Family services at ADAS but also between ADAS and statutory services such as the CDAT, as well as the child's school. Information was shared amongst the professionals working with the family and the mother and, where appropriate, with the child too. This enabled the mother to access the support she so badly needed, which, in turn, helped to ameliorate the home situation, thus making it a healthier environment, physically and emotionally, for both mother and son to live in.

*The names in the above example are fictitious and some details have been changed to protect the identity of the family involved.

As discussed earlier, even when difficulties are very pronounced, taking a whole-family approach can be beneficial.

Practice example 11, an example of the NSPCC's Family SMILES programme, explores working with families with mentally ill parents whose children are at risk of abuse or neglect.

Practice example 11: Family SMILES

Family SMILES (Simplifying Mental Illness + Life Enhancement Skills) is an adaptation of the Australian programme, SMILES, an evidence-based, young carer's, group-work model. SMILES was developed in 1997 by Erica Pitman as a result of the increasing recognition that children in families affected by mental illness are a population 'at risk' of developing their own mental health problems (Pitman 1997).

The NSPCC Family SMILES programme[17] is for families with mentally ill parents whose children are at risk of abuse or neglect. Family SMILES aims to boost children's self-esteem, enhance the parent's protective ability and improve the parent–child relationship through a whole-family approach.

Many parents with a mental illness care for their children satisfactorily, but in some cases parental mental illness can be responsible for serious interruptions in a child's cognitive and emotional development, which in turn can have implications for their future mental health. The negative effects of parental mental illness on children are not dependent on the parent's diagnosis but are related to that parent's behaviour, the responses of other key adults (both familial and professional) and the degree to which development of the child's resilience has been encouraged (Cooklin 2013).

Practice model

Family SMILES is a twin-track programme working with children and their parents.

NSPCC social workers deliver an eight-week group-work programme for children aged between 8 and 13 years for up to eight children to build self-esteem and provide education about mental health difficulties.

Work with the children is complemented by individual work with parents over six sessions to strengthen the parent–child relationship and improve parents' understanding of the impact of their illness on the child.

Throughout the course of the individual and group work, a bespoke safety plan is developed for the child so that should the child's parent become acutely ill, the child will be cared for safely. The responsibility for the child's safety will rest with adults, and the wishes of the child will be considered.

Evaluation

The evaluation of Family SMILES was designed by the NSPCC and commenced in 2010 across 8 sites and is now in 11 sites. The evaluation aims to find out whether children who have accessed the programme develop resilience and cope more effectively with living with parental mental illness and whether the parent–child relationship is improved.

Data is collected at three points from children, parents, practitioners and professionals who referred families using both quantitative and qualitative methods.

Evaluation tools include the Child Abuse Potential Inventory, The Child's Self-Esteem Scale based on Rosenberg and Goodman's SDQ (Strengths and

---

17   For further information, contact: Di Jerwood, NSPCC, Children's Services Development and Delivery, Families with Complex Needs, Tel: 07717 881735

Difficulties Questionnaire) and HoNOSCA (Health of the Nation Outcome Scales (Children and Adolescents)), which is undertaken with the practitioners.

The evaluation is due to be completed in December 2015; interim findings show that children who accessed Family SMILES had increased self-esteem and less serious emotional and behavioural problems. Parents reported increased self-esteem and lower levels of distress and unhappiness.

Both parents and children appreciated the opportunity to talk more openly about mental health issues and the impact on the family and to find some solutions.

Further evaluation will provide more insight into whether these changes were sustained in the longer term, as well as findings from a comparison group of parents and children who have not received the service.

Quotes from parents and children who have accessed the Family SMILES programme

I never really felt comfortable talking to my mum about anything. My mum is starting to tell me stuff, and usually before I would probably go: 'I don't really care.' But I do care now. (Young person)

I thought I was doing right by letting her deal with her own thing, when actually now she'll ask me for five minutes and we'll sit and talk. (Parent)

But I was able to talk to him then more about it and I learnt that from [Family] SMILES. It's OK to discuss things with your child and it's OK to say 'I'm not feeling well', which before I would have said nothing. Just 'Oh, mummy hurt her back today', or 'mummy tripped and fell', or something, I'd come up with these reasons for being in bed or if I'd been crying or whatever. Definitely, definitely made a big difference. (Parent with a severe mental health problem)

In this chapter we have explored in some detail the ways in which direct practice can be developed to support families better. As should have been apparent from earlier discussions in this handbook, this area of work is and will continue to be challenging. Using some of the ideas and approaches presented here to think creatively and keep a focus on the needs of the child and wider family, on building resilience and on developing the strengths and harnessing the resources of the family, wider community and informal and formal support networks should go some way towards helping practitioners improve assessments and the direct support they provide to children, parents and whole families including fathers.

6

What more can services do at the strategic level to support families more effectively?

This chapter looks beyond the immediate practice realm to examine what more services can do at a strategic level to provide effective services and practice to children and families affected by parental substance misuse and/or parental mental health difficulties. It considers a number of selected strategic-level considerations and interventions, which, in our view, are most likely to help practitioners respond to the barriers and concerns highlighted in Chapter 4. It looks at: user involvement; joint working culture and protocols; creating and promoting more accessible services including tackling stigma, addressing race and culture and developing father-inclusive services.

While this handbook is primarily focused on improving practice, it is generally accepted that practice operates in, and its effectiveness is contingent on, the wider strategic landscape and organisational culture. Critical to the development of effective practice will be the extent to which joint working culture is part of the agency vision and is actively promoted and pursued with visible and voluble support from those with authority and control of resources and with supportive systems, processes and structures in place.

Local strategic leaders and service managers need to make sure that the issues and impacts of parental substance misuse and parental mental health problems are not overlooked because of a lack of specifically targeted policies or initiatives. Additionally, they need to take steps to understand the full extent of the issues and their impacts, not only within their particular service domain but more widely across the wide range of systems and agencies, for children and adults including local health, public health, social care, crime and education agencies. Furthermore, strategic leaders need to make effective use of important tools such as the Joint Strategic Needs Assessment (JSNA) for cross-agency strategic engagement to improve the collecting, sharing and use of data to inform joint commissioning, planning and service delivery. Making sure that Health and Wellbeing Boards have the right representation and that the Health and Wellbeing Strategy fully reflects the needs and issues for these particular vulnerable families are also key. Leaders have to think creatively and laterally to make best use of high-profile initiatives and policy levers, such as crime reduction strategies, and of initiatives such as the Troubled Families programme and the Social Care Innovation programme. Research in Practice has produced a strategic prompt on parental substance misuse (Martins 2013), which includes a number of questions to consider when planning strategies to address parental substance misuse. A similar set of questions could be asked in relation to parental mental health.

Below we have selected some strategic issues to examine in a little more depth. This list is by no means exhaustive, but the issues are particularly salient to practice in these areas.

User involvement

Improving the effectiveness of parental and family support services depends on listening and responding to previous and current service users' experiences, views and ideas about those services. Statutory and voluntary services have increasingly become aware of the value, and indeed the necessity (if services are to be truly responsive), of enabling children's participation in decisions affecting them and in facilitating the involvement of service users in service development.

Where service users have been meaningfully involved, the benefits can be a greater sense of ownership of the services by users, greater engagement, increased accessibility and flexibility, improved communication and, not least, more effective services that are more likely to achieve their desired outcomes.

Service users can be involved in service provision on the macro level (for example in protocol development or helping map needs and gaps geographically across areas) or at the micro level (for example introducing more choice and involvement in individual packages of support, for individual users or families, including encouraging professional flexibility in terms of where workers meet clients).

However service users are involved, it is vital that there is clarity about the purpose and the expectations surrounding their involvement. Thought needs to be given to the level and resourcing of any support required and to making sure that when feedback is given, its effect is visible in concrete action. This is particularly important for these families, given that support needs and ambivalence are likely to be high and trust levels low. For parents with mental health and/or substance misuse difficulties, or for their children, involvement via groups should not be the only option available. Confidentiality will be a critical concern for them, so the availability of one-to-one opportunities might help to increase engagement. Also important are the usual practical considerations such as timing, access, help with transport and childcare and also, crucially, a neutral setting, avoiding for example, a setting where a child protection conference may have taken place.

When done well, service-user involvement adds meaning and value to a service. Whilst many organisations have 'user involvement' or 'participation workers' or commission these tasks from specialist agencies, it is important that responsibility for accessing and utilising service-user feedback is owned by everyone within a service. The user represents the service, and it is essentially everyone's responsiveness and openness that will determine how service users view the service – and therefore how inclined they will be to enter into a dialogue that occurs naturally and in an ongoing, more immediate way.

Joint working culture

As discussed in Chapters 1 and 4, joint working is an essential, yet hard-to-achieve goal. Among the longstanding barriers that get in the way are the financial constraints and separate eligibility thresholds that different services work to. These constraints have been particularly pronounced in recent years because of the wider economic climate. Martins (2013), in her discussion of the challenges of addressing parental substance misuse effectively in the face of significant funding pressures, argues that local areas need to:

> use high-profile levers such as crime reduction to drive forward progress in this area…For instance, drug treatment is critical to achieving local successes around reduction of crime and improving individual, family and well-being outcomes. Addressing parental substance misuse may also help turn around the lives of those families defined as 'troubled'.(p.5)

Visible and embedded commitment to joint working at all levels within and between both adults' and children's organisations is essential to developing a culture of joint working. Furthermore, regular and direct contact between professionals in different services is often a feature of services that are more successful in establishing whole-family approaches. Such contacts/meetings in various guises can be useful in: strengthening relationships; raising awareness; and improving coherence of systems and processes such as referral processes, joint visits, assessments and care plans.

Formal meetings, or for example attendance at referral meetings of other services, are only part of the picture. 'Getting about' by physically being in the same place and getting practitioners' faces, names and roles known across services also helps. Where staff know at least one person in a related service whom they feel able to access, collaboration is far more likely to occur and, most crucially, to occur at an earlier stage of intervention. Also, if workers are enabled and indeed expected to share their skills and knowledge and access each other's expertise – and supported in doing so by clear guidance and protocols as discussed below – this will improve their ability to respond holistically, confidently and appropriately to users' needs. Being able simply to 'have a chat' across service boundaries, even when thresholds for the other service are not met, is an essential part of preventative working and is supported by cultivating relationships with individuals.

SCIE has developed a range of resources on parental mental health and child welfare (including dual diagnosis) and provides good practice examples.[1]

Joint working protocols

Well-implemented joint working protocols can provide a foundation for establishing and cementing common working practices and can help to clarify expectations. They should provide clear instructions and requirements and be easy to use. SCIE, in its 2003 report *Families That Have Alcohol and Mental Health Problems: A Template for Partnership Working* (Kearney *et al.* 2003b), provides suggestions regarding protocol development and implementation. It stresses the need for protocols to arise from a collaboration between the relevant agencies, as this is a useful and necessary exercise in itself. To ensure that protocols are then implemented, they should be widely accessible and actively disseminated, backed up by launches and training, referred to regularly in supervision and practice development activities and included as an essential part of new workers' induction programmes. They also need to be regularly updated and their outcomes evaluated.

Improving interagency practice also requires the clear articulation of services' responsibilities and of mechanisms for challenging them when agencies fall down on fulfilling their responsibilities. Joint working protocols can help to bring clarity and to reduce misunderstanding between agencies. Also, involving service users as collaborators in the development of protocols provides a clear opportunity for them to influence services directly. To make sure that protocols remain live, helpful tools, it is also important that training and policy documents reference and underline their importance and that there are mechanisms for professionals and users to review their usefulness in practice and to refresh and update them as necessary.

Coherent policies e.g. on dual diagnosis

In Chapter 4 we discussed how dual diagnosis seems to be responded to at a service level with dual stigma, increased bureaucracy, delays and less efficiency. Clear guidance and policies regarding dual diagnosis are seen as helpful in addressing this; and national guidance on dual diagnosis does exist. In 2002 the Department of Health produced the *Mental Health Policy Implementation Guide: Dual Diagnosis Good Practice Guide* to provide a policy framework. Turning Point, a key organisation operating in the sector went on to produce a good practice handbook in 2007 in which they note that the Department of

---

1   www.scie.org.uk/atoz

Health guide provides 'a framework to help strengthen services and advocates a move towards an integrated system of care delivery'. They cite the guide's focus on:

> bringing the care of people with severe mental health problems and problematic substance use into the mainstream, through mental health services taking the primary responsibility for their treatment. (Turning Point 2007, p.2)

The intention, as Turning Point (2007) suggests is 'to avoid service users being shifted between services and falling through the net of care' (p.10).

> Guidance on good practice stresses the need for definitions to be agreed between agencies and for all relevant staff to be trained and equipped to work with dual diagnosis. There is also an emphasis on developing different models for inter-agency working including dedicated dual diagnosis teams and assertive outreach teams specialising in dual diagnosis. The need for clear expectations and arrangements between agencies links back to the need for joint working protocols, discussed earlier (Turning Point 2007).

Training and skills development

New developments such as Troubled Families programmes, Early Help programmes and initiatives such as the Social Care Innovation programme have triggered what appears to be a growth in the level and nature of multidisciplinary working. These new ways of working have generally been accompanied by an apparent upturn in joint training and development, especially in relation to engaging with ambivalent families and in developing a focus on outcomes. This is to be welcomed, and the learning, outcomes and impacts should be evaluated and used to inform future developments.

For these complex issues and agencies, alongside more traditional methods such as joint training, making formal arrangements for staff to visit and 'shadow' the work of other professionals or setting up secondments between services, can be very useful ways of enhancing the development of staff in both adults' and children's services. Thorough staff inductions that allow enough time for workers to get to grips with both their own organisation and the other relevant services (preferably through visits) are also important.

Training and development also need to integrate thinking around engaging with particular cohorts and groups that are not currently well served, such as fathers and some black and minority ethnic groups. It is also vital that skills and knowledge in relation to the needs of children are fully considered, and practice example 12 describes a process through which adult mental health workers identified and then addressed their training needs in this area.

Some resources for training and team development that may help enhance the knowledge, skills or awareness of professionals in their work with parental mental health or substance misuse are referred to in the Further Resources section.

Practice example 12 describes how adult mental health workers identified and addressed their knowledge and skills gaps through training in order to enable them to consider children's needs.

Practice example 12: Tower Hamlets
Home Treatment Team

This example explores how a Foundation Trust is breaking down barriers between adult mental health and children's services and helping a Home Treatment Team talk about parenting.

The multidisciplinary Home Treatment Team in Tower Hamlets, part of the East London Foundation Trust, has made significant strides in recognising the impact of mental illness on parenting and on children. This is in line with Trust policy on safeguarding children and raised expectations within the Trust that workers will not only identify risk to children, but also identify their wider emotional and developmental needs, while supporting the adults in their role as parents. This has led to some anxiety and questions from staff, who requested additional teaching input.

Staff identified their concerns and confusion about matters such as sharing information, making a referral to children and family services or routinely notifying children and family services of mental health services' involvement. These tasks created extra pressure for a team whose involvement with a family is likely to be brief. Disclosing information to another agency was thought to conflict with codes of practice and professional ethics.

The main anxiety seemed to lie in raising the matter at all with someone who may be very unwell. Staff were uncomfortable with the idea of telling a service user, who may be already acutely embarrassed by the need for mental health services' involvement, that they needed to inform or involve yet another agency. Staff were also unclear about whether there would be any benefit to the family of such actions.

The team invited the Coordinator for Children in Families with Mental Illness, who works across adults' mental health and children's services, to plan two workshops with them to help them find ways of managing these responsibilities in a way that they, as well as the service user, could feel comfortable with.[2]

For the first of these, the Coordinator invited the Trust's Safeguarding Children nurse advisor, and social workers from the Children and Families Advice and Assessment team, to clarify policy and referral procedures. The whole team participated in an informal quiz and had the opportunity to ask questions of the other service. Staff discovered that they knew more than they had previously thought, clarified points of confusion and became more realistic in

---

2   For further information, contact: Rosemary Loshak, Coordinator for Children in Families with Mental Illness, 7th Floor Anchorage House, 2 Clove Crescent, London E14 2BE, Email: Rosie.Loshak@towerhamlets.gov.uk or Lorette.McQueen@elcmht.nhs.uk

their expectations of the other service and respectful of each service's workloads. Differences of language, terminology and statutory framework were sorted out.

The second workshop focused on how to talk to families when one had concerns about children, and the Coordinator was joined by a CAMHS family therapist as co-facilitator. Through discussion and role-play, staff revealed deeper fears and anxieties but were also able to learn from each other and come up with a comprehensive list of good practice points.

Some of the fears expressed were about:

- facing the user's hostility
- breaking the therapeutic relationship and creating distrust
- increasing stigma
- impinging on civil liberties
- going against culturally prevalent behaviours – including what is appropriate in the worker's own culture
- making someone more ill by adding to existing stress
- creating fears that they would lose the children
- betraying the user
- obtaining 'permission to share information' then telling the whole world
- following procedure just because the political climate had changed.

Several workers reported that talking to families about the impact of the illness on their children was not a problem and, indeed, that to confront a client with the reality of the damage they might be causing to family relationships, and the likely consequences, could be a helpful therapeutic step.

The learning points that emerged from the discussion were that it was important to:

- feel clear and confident in your role and in what you are saying
- remain calm and matter of fact
- avoid jargon or legalistic language
- be transparent and fill in any forms together with the service user
- be positive about what might be gained from contacting children's services and from services working together
- recognise and acknowledge the support already available within the family
- pick up on the user's own concerns or wishes for help
- take care with timing and wait, unless there is an urgent situation, until the user's mental state allows them to listen and take in what is being said.

During the workshop, the team members were able to make positive use of their own varied experiences to identify good practice points and to learn from each other. There was increased confidence in what was possible and on the strengths of working together. Now participants are back at work, they report that they feel less anxious when discussing children's well-being with families and are able to present interventions in a more positive light. They have increased confidence when using their own initiative to liaise with schools and other children's services, with the families' agreement, and thinking about children is built into daily practice.

As stated in Chapter 4, as no one professional discipline can hold expertise or knowledge in all relevant aspects, better awareness of where and with whom expertise or knowledge is generally held and how to access it is essential. There is also a need for increased awareness and appreciation of the systemic nature of family functioning – the impact that one family member and their needs and behaviour has on another – as well as a clearer message within organisations that *supporting families* is everybody's responsibility.

> Combining the authority of senior managers and the dynamism of the voluntary sector and users is the most effective way of supporting staff seeking to put whole-family approaches into practice. Embedding the messages into induction, training, supervision and performance management can help promote the work, and altering assessment and recording tools, can prompt people to Think Family. (SCIE 2011, p.1)

SCIE also recommends the development of a 'Think Family Strategy'[3] to implement their guidance and that parents, children and carers are involved in all stages of development.

For more ideas and examples of developing and embedding whole-family approaches, see the SCIE resources.[4]

Creating and promoting more accessible services

As discussed in Chapter 4, a key barrier to effective support is the inaccessibility of services to users generally and to some groups such as fathers and black and minority ethnic groups in particular. The role of strategic leaders in addressing this and the insidious and persistent issue of stigma are discussed below.

Tackling stigma

There can be a tendency for stigma to be seen as something inevitable that cannot be changed (Thornicroft 2006). This view can understandably lead services to view it as out of their control and remit. However, the impacts on those affected who come into contact with services (or who don't come into contact but may need support) is very much within the remit of services. Supporting people in managing the impact on

---

3   www.scie.org.uk/publications/guides/guide30/summary.asp

4   www.scie.org.uk/publications/guides/guide30/puttingitintopractice/index.asp

them of stigma can help promote their overall well-being and recovery, is a vital part of any holistic assessment of needs and can help prevent difficulties from worsening and necessitating more extreme forms of intervention. Stigma and discrimination can affect people long after the symptoms of mental health problems have been resolved. Discrimination can lead to relapses in mental health problems and can intensify existing symptoms (Link *et al.* 1997).

As discussed earlier, the significance of discrimination and stigma continues to be marked, with some nine out of ten people affected by mental health problems experiencing discrimination with devastating impacts on their lives, including: feeling excluded from everyday activities; finding it harder to get or keep a job; feeling reluctant to seek help; making recovery slower; and affecting physical health (Time to Change Stigma Survey 2008). The stigma attached to drug use can also devastate lives, with dependent users and their families often delaying or not seeking help, fearing that once they do, they will be stuck with the label 'hopeless addict' for life and with professional attitudes all too often reinforcing stigma and lowering expectations of recovery (UKDPC 2010b).

There is a need for the relevant services not only to support people with the impact of stigma and discrimination, but also to ensure that services themselves are not the source of discrimination, treating people unfairly or denying them opportunities. A widespread recognition and adoption of a social model of disability is an important basis for change. Such a model reduces the tendency to locate the problem within the individual; instead it focuses on addressing disabling barriers, including negative attitudes and unequal access (Morris and Wates 2006). Currently, few interventions address the significant structural and social factors that affect the life outcomes for this group of families, despite previous research clearly identifying the need to do so (Fraser *et al.* 2006).

Ideas and resources for tackling stigma in services, workplaces and the wider community are available from initiatives such as Time to Change,[5] England's biggest programme to challenge mental health stigma and discrimination. Time to Change is seeking to empower people with mental health problems to feel confident talking about the issue without facing discrimination. The programme of activities being undertaken by Time to Change to help take forward this goal includes doing strategic work with organisations from all sectors to improve policy and practice around mental health discrimination. Initiatives to tackle stigma in relation to substance misuse are some way behind those targeting mental health but much can be learnt and transferred. The UKDPC (2010b) emphasises the necessity of tackling the stigmatisation of drugs dependence, which it sees as undermining any efforts to provide support to enable people to deal with and manage their condition and recovery, integration and rehabilitation. At minimum, those in charge of commissioning and running services should make sure that the way in which services are delivered does not add to the already considerable burden of stigma and that their staff are trained and developed to understand, tackle and provide help to alleviate the impacts.

---

5   www.time-to-change.org.uk

Addressing race and culture

The poor experiences and outcomes of black and minority ethnic groups in relation to mental health and substance misuse and the barriers and challenges to service and practice improvements are well documented, as outlined in Chapter 4. Increasing accessibility and service quality demands significant, strong, strategic-level leadership and support to create change throughout organisations. Engaging with communities and working with voluntary and community sector organisations and with users to develop responses are all part of the solution, as is learning and replicating lessons from elsewhere. For example, while the Strengthening Families, Strengthening Communities parenting programme run by the Race Equality Foundation is not specifically targeted at families in these particular circumstances, there is much that should be learnt from their experience and success in engaging parents from a range of backgrounds, including black and minority ethnic parents and parents from marginalised communities, including those with experience of drugs, alcohol or violence.

One approach to overcoming service barriers in order to meet the differing needs of black and minority ethnic families has involved trying to create an ethnically diverse workforce. This is a challenge for workforce development initiatives. Additionally, the existing workforce requires support in becoming more 'culturally capable' – as recommended by the Race Equality Action Plan. The current picture of race-related training is patchy and fragmented, with no agreed definition of 'cultural competence'. However, Joanne Bennet from the Sainsbury Centre for Mental Health (in Lyall 2006) found in her review of training that there is currently a lack of evidence that such race-related training works in producing better services. She argues that it is more important to look at structural processes and power relationships in the way services are delivered. Following the Lawrence inquiry, cultural competence training in the police had no effect according to Richard Stone (a panel member of the Lawrence and Bennet inquiries) (in Lyall 2006).

Training and awareness raising that is planned and delivered by or in conjunction with service users seems to be more effective. The East London and City Mental Health Trust held a focus group with service users, scriptwriters and staff and created a play to raise awareness of service user views, needs and experiences. Evaluation of the impact of this on the over 100 mental health staff who saw the play showed that they had an improved awareness of discrimination and many talked afterwards of the need to improve their listening skills as a result (Lyall 2006).

Another critical area for attention is meaningful engagement with users. Users' perspectives should be critical to needs analyses and to the plans and services that flow from them. As observed in the Race Equality Foundation *Better Health Briefing*:

Sustained and meaningful dialogue with both service providers and minority ethnic patients, carers and members of the public, can help to improve understanding of problems and find creative, viable solutions. (Lavis 2014, p.1)

Finally, strategic leaders and managers need to make sure that services are aware of and have the confidence to apply equality legislation and that they work hard to root out and tackle the dual and often multiple layers of stigma and discrimination attached to vulnerable black and minority ethnic families dealing with the complex challenges of parental substance misuse and/or parental mental health problems. They need good knowledge of The Equality Act 2010, which consolidated and replaced previous discrimination laws into one piece of legislation. Race and disability are among the nine protected characteristics[6] and people with such characteristics should not be discriminated against, either directly or indirectly. These are helpful and powerful levers, which services need to use more effectively.

Reaching fathers

The tendency for services to fail to include or engage with fathers successfully through assessment and provision of support services is well documented, as discussed in Chapter 4. When Ghate *et al.* (2000) looked at men's interactions with children's centre services they found that some of the positive factors that enabled men's involvement within such services were:

- referral-only centres or parts of centres – because men tended to stick more closely to programmes of involvement when they had formally been referred to centres (although some doubt existed as to whether fathers engaged with the centre in any more than a superficial way)

- management attitudes that were seen as objective, not biased towards mothers, and that involved actively encouraging fathers

- male workers (male facilitators of groups and activities were particularly important)

- a willingness of staff to build relationships with fathers on their own terms and often away from the family centre

- staff persistence

- referral systems targeted at both mothers and fathers

- a less hostile atmosphere – e.g. the presence of other men or male staff and a welcoming building

- activities that men saw as more 'male', such as those related to DIY, barbeques, parties and other types of social, family-oriented events.

---

6   Under the Equality Act 2010 particular groups are covered against discrimination as they have 'Protected characteristics'. There are nine of these: age, disability, gender reassignment, marriage or civil partnership, pregnancy or maternity, race, religion and belief, sex, and sexual orientation.

Some services, such as substance misuse services, are more experienced in working with men individually and in groups (Morris and Wates 2006). It is worth services that struggle with this finding out more about the structures and models of service provision that seem to be successful in engaging men. Family Group Conferences are another model within children's services that have been successful in involving fathers.

> It requires going out there because you have to overcome a cultural thing. A service to get there needs to be proactive. A lot of services say 'We are for everyone but fathers don't come.' It's the responsibility of the service. It's about targeting. There are lots of ways for targeting. It's where you market. Generally programmes find that you have to go to where the fathers are – you have to go to them – pubs, sports clubs, employers. Employment agencies. You have to organise activities that men feel comfortable with. (National Voluntary Organisation in Department for Education and Skills 2006b, p.33).

The critical importance of reaching men should not be underestimated; there is an urgent need for shifts in service culture and systems (as discussed in Chapter 4) in order that the potential risks and untapped resources of so-called 'hidden men' are considered. In a recent NSPCC review (NSPCC Information Service 2015) of serious case reviews published since 2008, two categories of hidden men emerged: men who posed a risk to the child that resulted in them suffering harm; and men, for example estranged fathers, who were capable of protecting and nurturing the child but were overlooked by professionals. Recommendations for managers included the need for supervisors 'to offer guidance and training on working with fathers and male carers, monitor fathers' engagement with services and evaluate how effective direct work with them is'(Community Care 2012).

In its top tips for managers, *Community Care* recommends that they:

- ensure safety plans are in place in every case that involves violent or threatening parents and consider a zero-tolerance approach
- commission high-quality perpetrator programmes that include a significant element of dealing with fatherhood
- change IT systems to ensure details of fathers are required
- ensure that all services, including early intervention, are meeting the needs of men as well as women
- foster better partnership working across commissioned services
- ensure all social workers have access to training or continuing professional development (CPD) that includes theories about masculinity, gender, cultural influences on masculinity and dealing with violent or threatening behaviour.

(Community Care 2012)

Some local areas, for example, Islington's Children in Need team, have been trialling new ways of working to improve engagement with fathers. This involves working on developing new processes and practice across teams and with other agencies.

In this chapter we have explored in some detail the ways in which strategic leaders and service managers can make sure that the services they oversee can be developed to better support families. An enabling strategic environment is essential for the development of creative, dynamic practice in this challenging area. This chapter has highlighted what can be done at the strategic level from developing joint working agreements and protocols between agencies, through joint training of staff and the development of policies and services which tackle stigma, challenge discrimination and operate inclusively to build user and community capacity and resilience. The ideas presented here should go some way towards helping practitioners and managers to improve the support and services provided to children, to parents and to whole families including fathers and to making sure that such services are accessible and non-stigmatising and reach the full diversity of users.

7
Final summary

Chapter 1 of this handbook highlighted that parental substance misuse and parental mental health problems affect a substantial portion of the population as a whole and in particular those who come into contact with services. There is an urgent and essential need for services to respond effectively to the needs of families affected by these issues, because while their presence does not necessarily result in adverse outcomes for children, it often does, and the impact on them can be serious and long-lasting.

An examination of the potential impact of such family circumstances on children in Chapter 2 demonstrates that there is a lack of research into families who are coping well and that most research is focused on mothers rather than fathers. The research that is available mainly concerns families who come into contact with services and illustrates that they have an increased likelihood of experiencing poverty, poor housing, stigma and isolation.

The ability of parents to ensure their children's safety and provide boundaries, stimulation, physical care, supervision, consistency and routines can be significantly impeded. For children, this can have a cumulative impact that is detrimental to their physical and mental health. They may develop emotional and behavioural difficulties and experience reduced integration and success in their education, and they may adopt coping strategies that are not necessarily positive. Many children become young carers, adding to the challenges they face and the sense of responsibility they may feel. Where parents struggle to show emotional warmth to their children due to their changing moods or presentation, this can affect children's self-esteem and ability to form relationships, as can the secrecy and stigma often experienced by children in these circumstances.

Less often, children can be at risk of abuse or serious neglect that could be fatal (for example where dangerous substances are accessible to children) or at least significantly harmful. There is increasing recognition of the impact of neglect on children of all ages including adolescents. At the same time, the potential risks to children can increase: for very young children or babies; when mental health problems are psychotic in nature or parental delusions involve the child; when domestic violence is present; or when substance misuse is coupled with mental ill health.

Broader research into 'resilience' (discussed in Chapter 3) indicates that the presence of certain 'protective factors' are associated with better outcomes and increased resilience for children and families. These protective factors include: a supportive partner; accessible and non-stigmatising community resources; a stable, trustworthy adult within or outside the extended family who takes a consistent interest in a child's life; supportive social networks; and the opportunity to achieve, build self-esteem and maintain important family rituals and routines.

In order to safeguard children and to support families in better meeting their needs, it is essential that professional responses are based both on a good understanding of the day-to-day experience of children and the actual or likely impact on the developing child of any specific unmet needs or risks that are present, alongside a good understanding of the family's experiences and needs. Generalisations and value judgements need to be guarded against and, where possible, the positive aspirations of family members, their motivation for change and their strengths need to be recognised and harnessed to support better outcomes. An increased understanding of the importance of protective factors among families, and the professionals who work with them, could empower people to influence and nurture the positives and strengths, perhaps leading to better outcomes.

If children cannot safely remain within their immediate family, timely and robust decisions need to made about their future. This should be based on a sound understanding of individual circumstances and a thorough exploration of whether or not the provision of appropriate support could ameliorate the situation within the timescale appropriate to the child's needs. Throughout this handbook the point has been made that the provision of appropriate support is sometimes lacking and there is often scope for professional responses to be more focused, coordinated and therefore more effective.

There are a number of reasons for this. Relevant legislation and policy (discussed in Chapter 1 and the Appendix) has tended to be fragmented, often failing to recognise adult service users as parents and the impact that individual family members have on one another. Furthermore, the structure of 'single-user' services militates against a 'family focus'. Resource constraints lead to high thresholds for services and limited support being on offer. As a result, despite the goodwill and rhetoric about preventive services and more integrated working, statutory services continue, all too often, to be reactive, inaccessible and not joined up in their approach. Outcomes for families are poor, with only half of 'problem drug-using' parents known to services having their children still living with them. Interventions tend to occur late and at 'the heavy end'. For the many more children adversely affected by parental alcohol use there is a tendency for under-intervention or for significant delays in decision-making. For those affected by parental mental health problems, there is little support when mental health problems are classed as 'mild' or 'moderate' even though the impact on the child can still be significant.

Other hindrances to good practice in this area were discussed in Chapter 4. They indicate a need for more collaborative, analytical assessments and decision-making and an increase in knowledge and awareness among adults' and children's practitioners. Other obstacles include the challenge of engaging with resistant service users or those who fear services, along with practical barriers, for example a lack of family-friendly facilities within traditionally 'adult' services such as psychiatric hospitals or drug services.

Chapter 5 explored some of the ways in which practice can better support families. It included the need for: training and skills development; assessments that are clear, focus on the child as well as the wider family and are informed by research and theory; focused, whole-family support (including support to children; parents – fathers as well as mothers; and the family as a whole) that is strengths based and is helpful to children and parents practically and emotionally. Chapter 6 then gave consideration to those things that could be done at a more strategic level to bring about improvements. To enable relevant professionals to 'think family', there needs to be a clear message coming from senior levels of organisations that safeguarding children is everybody's responsibility. This needs to be supported by clear expectations about working, backed up by protocols, training and coherent policies in related areas such as dual diagnosis and kinship care. Organisations need to be proactive in increasing the accessibility of their services by reducing stigma and making them more relevant and appealing to black and minority ethnic families, to fathers and to other potential service users who may anticipate that services will be discriminatory towards them.

An examination of the practice and strategic barriers and the changes necessary to enable services to better respond to parental mental health or parental substance misuse illustrates a much wider issue. There is a need for more integrated, family-focused services across the board, in all circumstances where individual needs impact on families as a whole. It is likely that many suggestions about strategic and practice issues made within this handbook will be relevant to working with other families with complex needs.

Finally, it is important to acknowledge that there is much good work already being undertaken with individuals and with families, and there is a wealth of knowledge, skills and positive motivation within the children's and adults' services workforce. To support this further, a culture of collaboration and joint working, even informally 'picking each other's brains' when thresholds are not met, along with an openness to learn from each other and from service users, can only be beneficial for service users and practitioners alike.

Further resources

Below is an alphabetical list of relevant organisations and website addresses that are sources of additional relevant information. A few relevant books, videos and training packages are also listed.

Organisations and their websites
Adfam

www.adfam.org.uk

Provides telephone advice, website information and services for families affected by alcohol and drug misuse. It has also produced the following publications:

Bouncing Back!

Creative learning pack for work with families, available from Adfam website, price £15.

We Count Too

Published by three family-support organisations: Adfam, Pada and Famfed.

These are good practice guides for those working with family members affected by someone else's drug use: www.adfam.org.uk/professionals/reference_and_research/ adfam_publications/we_count_too

Adfam
25 Corsham Street
London N1 6DR
Tel: 020 7553 7640
Fax: 020 7253 7991

Email: admin@adfam.org.uk

Alcohol Concern

www.alcoholconcern.org.uk

Provides information on services, factsheets on alcohol, and a helpline.

Alcohol Concern
Suite B5 West Wing
New City Cloisters
196 Old Street
London EC1V 9FR
Tel: 020 7566 9800

Barnardo's

www.barnardos.org.uk

Produces publications, including free downloads, practitioner resources, young carers' projects and more.

Barnardo's
Tanners Lane
Barkingside
Ilford
Essex IG6 1QG
Tel: 020 8550 8822
Fax: 020 8551 6870

BASW

http://basw.co.uk/special-interest-groups/alcohol-and-other-drugs

Has a range of downloadable 'pocket guides' and resources relating to social work with families affected by substance use and alcohol. Among the numerous useful resources on offer is the *Pocket Guide for Social Workers on Mental Health and Substance Use* (Galvani and Livingstone 2012).

Tel: 0121 622 3911

Care Quality Commission

www.cqc.org.uk

Runs a website that includes information for service users, carers, children and professionals. Information is available in different languages.

CQC National Customer Service Centre
Citygate
Newcastle NE1 4PA
Tel: 03000 616161

The Centre for Excellence and Outcomes in Children and Young People's Services (C4EO)

www.c4eo.org.uk

Provides a range of products and support services to improve outcomes. For the first time, excellence in local practice, combined with national research and data about 'what works' is being gathered in one place. C4EO shares this evidence and the best of local practice with all those who work with and for children and young people and provides practical, 'hands-on support' to help local areas make full use of this evidence. One of its key work themes is 'Families, parents and carers – improving the safety, health and well-being of children through improving the physical and mental health of mothers, fathers and carers.'

C4EO
8 Wakley Street
London EC1V 7QE
Switchboard: 020 7843 6358
Email: contactus@c4eo.org.uk

Centre for Mental Health

www.centreformentalhealth.org.uk

Works to improve quality of life for people with mental health problems by influencing policy and practice in mental health services. The focus is mainly on criminal justice and employment, and broad mental health policy. The aims of the Centre are furthered through project work, research, publications and events.

The Centre for Mental Health
Maya House
134–138 Borough High Street
London SE1 1LB
Tel: 020 7827 8300
Fax: 020 7827 8369
Email: contact@centreformentalhealth.org.uk

ChildLine

www.childline.org.uk

The free national helpline for children and young people in danger and distress. It provides a confidential counselling service for any child with any problem 24 hours a day, every day. It listens, comforts and protects. Trained counsellors provide support and advice and can refer children in danger to appropriate helping agencies.

NSPCC
Weston House
42 Curtain Road
London EC2A 3NH
Helpline: 0800 1111

The Children's Society

www.childrenssociety.org.uk

Supports the STARS Project, a national initiative providing information and support for children and young people whose parents misuse drugs/alcohol.

www.starsnationalinitiative.org.uk

STARS Project, Tel: 0115 942 2974

Children of Addicted Parents and People

www.coap.co.uk

A self-help website for young people to discuss their concerns about a person who is abusing drugs or alcohol.

Community Care Inform

www.ccinform.co.uk

A range of guides for practitioners and managers including guides on engaging fathers.

Dartington Social Research Unit

www.dartington.org.uk

Undertakes and reports on research regarding children in need, child development and children's services.

Dartington Social Research Unit
Lower Hood Barn
Dartington
Devon TQ9 6AB

Tel: 01803 762400
Fax: 01803 762983
Email: unit@dartington.org.uk

Department for Education

www.education.gov.uk

Information includes research, statistics and data for professionals and families.

Department for Education
Castle View House
East Lane
Runcorn
Cheshire WA7 2GJ

Tel: 0370 0002288
Typetalk: 18001 0370 0002288 (contact also through website)

Department of Health

www.dh.gov.uk

Provides health and social care policy, guidance and publications. Information about alcohol misuse and substance misuse can be accessed on this site.

Department of Health
Richmond House
79 Whitehall
London SW1A 2NS

Tel: 020 7210 4850
Text phone: 020 7210 5025

Disabled Parents Network

www.disabledparentsnetwork.org.uk

Produces reports and guidance for professionals and handbooks to support disabled parents, their families and those working with them.

Tel: 08717 300 103

Email: information@disabledparentsnetwork.org.uk

DrugScope

www.drugscope.org.uk

An independent centre of expertise on drugs, informing policy development and reducing drug-related risk. The website includes information and drug data database of drugs literature. The information is available in different languages. 'D World' is a drug-information website for 11–14-year-olds.

DrugScope
4th Floor
Asra House
1 Long Lane
London SE1 4PG

Telephone: 020 7234 9730
Fax: 020 7234 9773
Email: info@drugscope.org.uk

Families Anonymous

www.famanon.org.uk

Runs advice and support groups for families and friends who are concerned about the use of drugs or related behavioural problems. Literature also available.

Families Anonymous
Doddington and Rollo Community Association
Charlotte Despard Avenue
Battersea
London SW11 5HD

Helpline: 0845 1200 660
Tel: 0207 4984 680
Email: office@famanon.org.uk

Family Action

www.family-action.org.uk

Provides home and project support for families, community-based mental health services and financial help for families. The website includes downloadable leaflets on services.
Family Action Head Office
24 Angel Gate
City Road
London EC1V 2PT

Tel: 020 7254 6251
Email: info@family-action.org.uk

Family Rights Group

www.frg.org.uk

Provides advice and support for families whose children are involved with social services, and develops and promotes services that help secure the best possible futures for children and families. Has information on family and friends as carers and on family group conferencing. Has a range of publications, including ones aimed at and about kinship carers. Information on Family Group Conferences (FGC) for policy makers, family members, managers, social workers, coordinators and anyone who may refer a family to, or attend, a FGC.

Family Rights Group
Second Floor
The Print House
18 Ashwin Street
London E8 3DL

Tel: 020 7923 2628
Fax: 020 7923 2683
Email: office@frg.org.uk
Advice Line: 0808 8010366
Advice Line: advice@frg.org.uk

Fatherhood Institute

www.fatherhoodinstitute.org

Describes itself as a 'think and do tank'. Produces materials and resources and provides training, consultancy for children and family services, schools and other agencies to help them become more father-inclusive. This includes materials for work with vulnerable families.

Fatherhood Institute
Unit 1
Warren Courtyard
Savernake
Marlborough
Wiltshire SN8 3UU

Tel: 0845 634 1328
Email: mail@fatherhoodinstitute.org

FRANK

www.talktofrank.com

A cross-departmental campaign led by the Department of Health/Home Office. Provides information and free confidential advice services through a helpline, and information and advice about drugs, their consequences and supporting services through a website and other resources.

Tel: 0300 123 6600 (24 hour)
SMS: 82111 (for texts)

Getting It Right For Every Child (GIRFEC)

www.gov.scot/Topics/People/Young-People/gettingitright/resources

The overarching framework for the Scottish Government, which works for children, young people and families. GIRFEC is being threaded through all existing policy, practice, strategy and legislation affecting children, young people and their families. Resources to support this work are available on the website.

Joseph Rowntree Foundation

www.jrf.org.uk

A social policy research and development charity. Its research themes include: housing, poverty, families, drugs and alcohol and mental health. Website includes publications.

JRF (Head Office)
The Homestead
40 Water End
York YO30 6WP

Tel: 01904 629241
Email: info@jrf.org.uk

Lifeline

www.lifeline.org.uk

Provides services for individuals and families affected by drug/alcohol misuse. Produces a range of publications about drugs and drug use.

Head Office
Lifeline Project Ltd
39–41 Thames St
Manchester M4 1NA

Tel: 0161 200 5486
Email: enquiries.lifeline@gmail.com

Mind

www.mind.org.uk

A mental health charity covering England and Wales. It is involved in:

- advancing the views, needs and ambitions of people with mental health problems
- challenging discrimination and promoting inclusion
- influencing policy through campaigning and education
- inspiring the development of quality services that reflect expressed need and diversity
- achieving equal rights through campaigning and education.

Tel: 0300 1233393 (information line)
Email: info@mind.org.uk

M-PACT

www.actiononaddiction.org.uk

The programme supports children/young people aged 8–17 who are experiencing the effects of parental substance misuse within the family. The programme offers a whole-family approach, working with parents and children from up to eight families at any one time in different group combinations.

Action on Addiction
Head Office
East Knoyle
Salisbury
Wilts SP3 6BE

Switchboard: 0300 330 0659
Fax: 01747 832028
Email: admin@actiononaddiction.org.uk

Nacro

www.nacro.org.uk

A crime reduction charity that aims to make society safer by finding practical solutions to reducing crime. Since 1966 Nacro has worked to give ex-offenders, disadvantaged people and deprived communities the help they need to build a better future.

Head office
NACRO
First Floor
46 Loman Street
London
SE1 0EH

Tel: 0300 123 1889
Fax: 020 7902 5448
Info and advice for families: Tel: 0300 123 1999
Email: helpline@nacro.org.uk

National Association for Children of Alcoholics (NACOA)

www.nacoa.org.uk

Founded to provide information, advice and support for children of alcoholics and people concerned for their welfare. Leaflets for children and parents are available as downloads.

Tel: 0800 358 3456 (a free confidential helpline)

Email: helpline@Nacoa.org.uk

National Children's Bureau (NCB)

www.ncb.org.uk

The National Children's Bureau is a leading research and development charity working to improve the lives of children and young people, reducing the impact of inequalities. NCB works with children, for children to influence government policy, be a strong voice for young people and front-line professionals, and provide practical solutions on a range of social issues.

Provides information on policy, research and best practice for professionals. The website includes information on publications (some downloadable) and current projects.

National Children's Bureau (NCB)
8 Wakley Street
London
EC1V 7QE

Tel: 020 7843 6000
Fax: 020 7278 9512

National Treatment Agency for Substance Misuse (NTA)

www.nta.nhs.uk

A special health authority, created by the government in 2001, to improve the availability, capacity and effectiveness of treatment for drug misuse in England. It is there to ensure that there is more treatment, better treatment and fairer treatment available to all those who need it. The website includes details of the NTA's work programme, as well as publications and guidance for those in the drug treatment sector and service users. Since 2013 the NTA has become part of Public Health England (PHE).

PHE Drugs, Alcohol, and Tobacco Team
2nd Floor
Skipton House
80 London Road
London SE1 6LH

Tel: 020 3682 0503
Email: enquiries@phe.gov.uk

Participation Works

www.participationworks.org.uk

Participation Works enables organisations to involve children and young people effectively in the development, delivery and evaluation of services that affect their lives. It is an online gateway to the world of children and young people's participation. The gateway provides a single access point to comprehensive information on policy, practice, networks, training and innovative ideas from across the UK.

Participation Works
C/O British Youth Council
49–51 East Road
London N1 6AH

Race Equality Foundation

www.raceequalityfoundation.org.uk

The Race Equality Foundation (formerly known as the Race Equality Unit) promotes race equality in social support (what families and friends do for each other) and public services (what 'workers' do with people who need support. It does this by: exploring what is known about discrimination and disadvantage; developing evidenced-based better practice to promote equality; disseminating better practice through educational activities, conferences, written material and websites. It has offices in London, Manchester and Leeds.

London office
Unit 17 & 22
Deane House Studios
27 Greenwood Place
London NW5 1LB

Tel: 0207 428 1880
Fax: 0207 428 0912

Research in Practice

www.rip.org.uk

The largest children and families research implementation project in England and Wales. Established in 1996, it is a department of The Dartington Hall Trust and is run in collaboration with the Association of Directors of Children's Services, The University of Sheffield and a network of over 100 participating agencies in the UK.

Its aims are to improve outcomes for vulnerable children and families in England and Wales by promoting and facilitating evidence-informed practice. The website provides news, views, research reviews, summaries, policy insights and information on projects and publications.

Research in Practice Social Justice Programme
The Granary
Dartington Hall
Totnes
Devon TQ9 6EQ

Tel: 01803 867692
Email: ask@rip.org.uk

Royal College of Psychiatrists

www.rcpsych.ac.uk

The professional and educational body for psychiatrists in the United Kingdom and the Republic of Ireland. It aims to promote mental health by: setting standards and promoting excellence in mental health care; improving understanding through research and education; leading, representing, training and supporting psychiatrists; and working with patients, carers and their organisations. The website includes information on drugs/ alcohol and mental illness.

The Royal College of Psychiatrists
21 Prescot Street
London
E1 8BB

Tel: 020 7235 2351
Tel: 020 7977 6655
Fax: 0203 701 2761
Email: reception@rcpsych.ac.uk

Social Care Institute for Excellence (SCIE)

www.scie.org.uk

Aims to improve the experience of people who use social care by developing and promoting knowledge about good practice in the sector. Using knowledge gathered from diverse sources and a broad range of people and organisations, it develops resources that are shared freely, supporting those working in social care and empowering service users. Its publications include:

SCIE Resource Guide 1: Families that have Alcohol and Mental Health Problems: A Template for Partnership Working. Available at: www.scie.org.uk/publications/resourceguides/rg01. pdf, accessed on 24 August 2015.

SCIE Report No 2. Alcohol Drug and Mental Health Problems: Working with Families. Available at: www.scie.org.uk/publications/reports/report02.pdf, accessed on 24 August 2015.

e-Learning Parental Substance Misuse. Available at: www.scie.org.uk/publications/ elearning/parentalsubstancemisuse, accessed on 24 August 2015.

Social Care Institute for Excellence
206 Marylebone Road
London NW1 6AQ

Tel: 020 7535 0900
Fax: 020 7535 090
Email: info@scie.org.uk

Start in Manchester (Startmc)

www.startmc.org.uk

An arts and mental health project. Its website provides information about the project and online art from adults with mental health issues. Startmc helps people to improve, maintain and protect their mental well-being through art and gardening. Service users are people recovering from a period of serious and long-term mental ill health, who want to use art to build confidence, self-esteem and practical life skills.

High Elms
Upper Park Road
Victoria Park
Manchester M14 5RU

Tel: 0161 257 0675 / 0161 257 0510 / 0161 257 0696
Fax: 0161 225 9410

Stella Project

www.avaproject.org.uk / our-projects / stella-project.aspx

The Stella Project addresses the overlapping issues of domestic and sexual violence, drug and alcohol use and mental health. They work for positive, sustained improvement in the way services are delivered to survivors, their children and perpetrators.

The Stella Project provides briefings, good practice guidance and toolkits.

For Stella Project enquiries contact:
Shabana Kausar or Lucy Allwright
0207 5490 275 or 0207 5490 255
shabana.kausar@avaproject.org.uk
lucy.allwright@avaproject.org.uk

Substance Misuse Management in General Practice (SMMGP)

www.smmgp.co.uk

A network to support GPs and other members of the primary healthcare team who work with substance misuse.

SMMGP
Box 200
143 Kingston Road
London SW19 1LJ

Email: smmgp@btinternet.com/admin@smmgp.org.uk

Time to Change

www.time-to-change.org.uk

Led by Mind and Rethink Mental Illness, Time to Change is England's largest programme aiming to tackle mental health stigma and discrimination.

Women's Aid

www.womensaid.org.uk

Provides information and help, including a 24-hour, national domestic violence helpline.

Women's Aid
PO Box 3245
Bristol BS2 2EH

Helpline: 0808 200 0247 / helpline@womensaid.org.uk
Tel: 0117 944 4411 (general enquiries only)
Fax: 0117 924 1703
Email: info@womensaid.org.uk

Books

Marge Heegaard (1993) *When a Family is in Trouble: Children can Cope with Grief from Drug and Alcohol Addiction*. Bloomington, MN: Woodland Press. ISBN: 978-0-96205-027-5.

Marge Heegaard (1991) *When Someone has a Very Serious Illness: Children can Learn to Cope with Loss and Change (Drawing Out Feelings)*. Bloomington, MN: Woodland Press. ISBN: 978-0-96205-024-4.

Evelyn Leite and Pamela Espeland (1999) *Different Like Me: A Book for Teens who Worry about their Parent's Use of Alcohol/Drugs*. Center City, MN: Hazelden Information and Educational Services. ISBN: 978-0-93590-834-3.

Pamela L. Higgins (1994) *Up and Down the Mountain: Helping Children Cope with Parental Alcoholism*. Liberty Corner, NJ: New Horizons Press. ISBN: 978-0-88282-133-7.

NCB publications

Available to purchase on the Jessica Kingsley Publishers website: www.jkp.com

Butcher, J. and Ryan, M. (2006) *Talking About Alcohol and Other Drugs: A Guide for Looked After Children's Services*. ISBN: 978-1904787785.

For managers of looked-after children's services, training managers, managers of children's and young people's residential homes and social workers.

Hart, D. and Powell, J. (2007) *Adult Drug Problems, Children's Needs: Assessing the Impact parental drug use – a Toolkit for Practitioners.* ISBN: 978-1-90478-797-6.

Provides a range of practice tools including checklists for: 'engagement and assessment', 'team managers', 'thinking about care planning' (which refers to when residential family placements should be considered, the need for plans to reflect children's needs and timescales, and twin-track planning) and 'supporting kinship carers'; and provides a checklist to use when 'considering a specialist assessment' and for 'suggestions for foster carers'.

Also includes a model for assessment, training tools and forms for auditing social work practice and for reviewing multi-agency working.

For more information on any of NCB's publications email publications@ncb.org.uk.

Training and development resources
Crossing Bridges

This publication provides comprehensive training for staff working with mentally ill parents and their children. Commissioned by the Department of Health, this training resource has been designed to enhance practice and improve services for families in which mentally ill adults live together with dependent children. The training manual aims to improve individual practice whilst encouraging interagency collaboration across specialist areas. The key approach of the training works on the premise that children and their mentally ill parents are better supported and protected if agencies coordinate services and interventions.

Falkov, A., Mayes, K. and Diggins, M. (1999) *Crossing Bridges.* Brighton: Pavilion Publishing. ISBN: 978-1-90060-048-4.

Keeping the Family in Mind

The Keeping the Family in Mind project undertaken by Barnardo's has produced an information pack and a video made by young carers whose parents have experienced mental health problems. It is a useful resource for professionals, including those working in adult mental health and children and families professionals. For further details, contact:

Barnardo's Action with Young Carers
24 Colquitt Street
Liverpool
L1 4DE

Tel: 0151 708 7323

www.barnardos.org.uk/keeping_the_family_in_mind.pdf

Being Seen and Heard

This training pack from the Royal College of Psychiatrists comprises a DVD/video with a CD-ROM of additional resources and a copy of the Royal College of Psychiatrists' report *Patients as Parents* (2002). The training film has been developed for the use of staff involved in the care of mentally ill parents and their children – whether from the health, social care, education, probation or voluntary sector services.

Part I shows children and parents relating their various experiences of the referral process.

Part II focuses on solutions and the ways in which professionals can help. The stories are interspersed with comments from experts.

The parents and children who have contributed to the film have given their permission on the strict understanding that the film will be used for training purposes only.

www.rcpsych.ac.uk/publications/books/rcpp/1904671438.aspx

References

Abdulrahim, D. (2006) 'Black and Minority Ethnic Drug Use.' In D. Hart, and J. Powell (eds) *Adult Drug Problems, Children's Needs: Assessing the Impact of Parental Drug Use – A Toolkit for Practitioners*. London: National Children's Bureau.

ACMD (Advisory Council on the Misuse of Drugs) (2003) *Government Response to Hidden Harm: The Report of an Inquiry by the Advisory Council on the Misuse of Drugs*. London: Department for Education and Skills.

ACMD (Advisory Council on the Misuse of Drugs) (2011) *Hidden Harm: Report of the Findings of the ACMD's Inquiry on Children of Problem Drug Users in the UK*. London: Home Office.

Adamson, J. and Templeton, L. (2012) *Silent Voices: Supporting Children and Young People Affected by Parental Alcohol Misuse*. London: The Office of the Children's Commissioner.

Aldridge, T. (1999) 'Family values: Rethinking children's needs living with drug abusing parents.' *Druglink* March/April, 8–11.

Aldridge, J. and Becker, S. (2003) *Children Who Care for Parents with Mental Illness: The Perspectives of Young Carers, Parents and Professionals*. Bristol: Policy Press.

Bancroft, A., Wilson, S., Cunningham-Burley, S., Backett-Milburn, K. and Masters, H. (2004) *Parental Drug and Alcohol Misuse: Resilience and Transition Among Young People*. York: Joseph Rowntree Foundation.

Barnard, M. A. and Barlow, J. (2003) 'Discovering parental drug dependence: silence and disclosure.' *Children and Society* 17, 1, 45–56.

Bates, T., Buchanan, J. and Corby, B. (1999) *Drug Use, Parenting and Child Protection: Towards an Effective Interagency Response*. Preston: University of Central Lancashire.

Bee, H. (2000) *The Developing Child*. Needham Heights, MA: Allyn and Bacon.

Bennett, G. (1989) *Treating Drug Abusers*. London: Routledge.

Bostock, L., Bairstow, S., Fish, S. and McCleod, S. (2005) *Managing Risks and Minimising Mistakes in Services to Children and Families* (SCIE Report 6). London: Social Care Institute for Excellence.

Bostock, L., Bairstow, S., Fish, S. and McCleod, S. (2005) *Managing Risks and Minimising Mistakes in Services to Children and Families* (SCIE Report 6). London: SCIE.

Brandon, M., Sidebotham, P., Bailey, S. and Belderson, P. (2011) *A Study of Recommendations Arising from Serious Case Reviews 2009–2010*. London: Department for Education.

Sidebotham, P., Bailey, S., Belderson, P., Hawley, C., Ellis, C. and Megson, ., *New Learning From Serious Case Reviews: A Two-year Report for 2009–2011.* ...on: Department for Education, Centre for Research on the Child and Family in the School of Social Work and Psychology, University of East Anglia Health Sciences Research Institute, Medical School, University of Warwick.

Brisby, T., Baker, S. and Hedderwick, T. (1997) *Under the Influence: Coping with Parents who Drink Too Much. A Report on the Needs of Children and Problem Drinking Parents.* London: Alcohol Concern.

Broadhurst, K., White, S., Fish, S., Munro, E., Fletcher, K. and Lincoln, H. (2010) *Ten Pitfalls and How to Avoid Them: What Research Tells Us.* London: NSPCC.

Burti, L., Amddeo, F., Ambros, M., Bonetto, C. *et al.* (2005) 'Does additional care provided by a consumer self-help group improve psychiatric outcome? A study in Italian community-based psychiatric service.' *Community Mental Health Journal 41*, 6, 705–720.

Cabinet Office, Social Exclusion Taskforce (2008) *Think Family: Improving the Life Chances of Families at Risk.* London: Cabinet Office.

Cade, B. and O'Hanlon, W. H. (1993) *A Brief Guide to Brief Therapy.* New York: WW Norton.

Calder, M. C. and Hackett, S. (eds) (2003) *Assessment in Childcare: Using and Developing Frameworks for Practice.* Lyme Regis: Russell House Publishing.

Care Quality Commission (2011) *Count Me in 2010. Results of the 2010 National Census of Inpatients and Patients on Supervised Community Treatment in Mental Health and Learning Disability Services in England and Wales.* Care Quality Commission and National Mental Health Development Unit.

Cleaver, H., Unell, I. and Aldgate, J. (1999) *Children's Needs, Parenting Capacity: The Impact of Parental Mental Illness, Problem Alcohol and Drug Use, and Domestic Violence on Children's Development.* London: Department of Health and The Stationery Office.

Cleaver, H., Unell, I. and Aldgate, J. (2011) *Children's Needs, Parenting Capacity: The Impact of Parental Mental Illness, Problem Alcohol and Drug Use, and Domestic Violence On Children's Development* (2nd ed.). London: The Stationery Office.

Community Care (2012) 'What about Dad? Why social workers need to know more about gender and masculinity.' *Community Care,* 4 May.

Cooklin A. (2013) 'Promoting children's resilience to parental mental illness: engaging the child's thinking.' *Advances in Psychiatric Treatment 19*, 3, 229–240.

Corrigan, P. W. (ed.) (2004) *On the Stigma of Mental Illness: Practical Strategies for Research and Social Change.* Washington, DC: American Psychological Association.

Dalzell, R. and Sawyer, E. (2007) *Putting Analysis into Assessment: Undertaking Assessments of Need – A Toolkit for Practitioners* (1st ed.). London: National Children's Bureau.

Dalzell, R. and Sawyer, E. (2011) *Putting Analysis into Assessment: Undertaking Assessments of Need – A Toolkit for Practitioners* (2nd ed.). London: NCB.

Dalzell, R. and Sawyer, E. (2016) *Putting Analysis into Child and Family Assessment: Undertaking Assessments of Need – A Toolkit for Practitioners.* London: Jessica Kingsley Publishers.

Daniel, B., Wassell, S., Gilligan, R. and Howe, D. (2010) *Child Development for Child Care and Child Protection Workers.* London: Jessica Kingsley Publishers.

Department for Education (2011) *The Munro Review of Child Protection Final Report: A Child-centred System.* London: Department for Education.

Department for Education and Skills (2006a) *Parenting Support: Guidance for Local Authorities in England.* London: Department for Education and Skills.

Department for Education and Skills (2006b) *Children's Services: The Market for Parental and Family Support Services.* London: Department for Education and Skills.

Department of Health (2000) *Framework for the Assessment of Children in Need and their Families: Family and Environmental Factors, Parenting Capacity and Children's Developmental Needs.* London: The Stationery Office.

Department of Health (2002) *Mental Health Policy Implementation Guide: Dual Diagnosis Good Practice Guide.* London: Department of Health.

Department of Health (2003) *Delivering Race Equality: A Framework for Action.* London: Department of Health.

Department of Health (2012) *No Health without Mental Health. Mental Health Strategy Implementation Framework Guidance.* London: HM Government.

Diggins, M., Constant, H., Roscoe, H. and Ewart-Boyle, S. (2011) *Think Child, Think Parent, Think Family: A Guide to Parental Mental Health and Child Welfare.* London: SCIE.

Edwards, R. and Gillies, V. (2005) *Resources in Parenting: Access to Capitals Project Report.* London: University of South Bank, Families and Social Capital, ESRC Research Group.

Elliot, E. and Watson, A. (1998) *Fit To Be A Parent: The Needs of Drug Using Parents in Salford and Trafford.* Manchester: Manchester Public Health and Research Centre, University of Salford.

Ericksen, J. R. and Henderson, A. D. (1992) 'Witnessing family violence: The children's experience.' *Journal of Advanced Nursing 17*, 1200–1209.

Fahlberg, V. M. D. (1991) *A Child's Journey Through Placement.* Indianapolis, IN: Perspectives Press.

Falkov, A. (ed.) (1998) *Crossing Bridges: Training Resources for Working with Mentally Ill Parents and their Children. Reader for Managers, Practitioners and Trainers.* London: Department of Health.

Fatherhood Institute and Family Rights Group (2012) *Engaging with Men in Social Care: A Good Practice Guide.* Wiltshire: Fatherhood Institute and Family Rights Group.

Fatherhood Institute (2013) *Engaging with Men in Social Care: A Good Practice Guide.* Marlborough: Fatherhood Institute and Family Rights Group.

Fish, S., Munro, E. and Bairstow, S. (2008) *Learning Together to Safeguard Children: Developing a Multi-agency Systems Approach for Case Reviews.* London: Social Care Institute for Excellence.

Fonagy, P., Steele, M., Steele, H., Higgitt A. and Target, M. (1994) 'The theory and practice of resilience.' *Journal of Child Psychology and Psychiatry 35*, 2, 231–257.

Forrester, D. (2000) 'Parental substance misuse and child protection in a British sample: A survey of children on the child protection register in an inner-London district office.' *Child Abuse Review 9*, 4, 235–246.

Forrester, D. (2004) 'Social Work Assessments with Parents Who Misuse Drugs or Alcohol.' In R. Phillips *Children Exposed to Parental Substance Misuse: Implications for Family Placement.* London: BAAF.

Forrester, D. (2012) *Parenting a Child Affected by Parental Substance Misuse.* London: BAAF.

Forrester, D. and Harwin, J. (2006) 'Parental substance misuse and child care social work: Findings from the first stage of a study of 100 families.' *Child and Family Social Work 11*, 4, 325–335.

Forrester, D., McCambridge, J., Waissbein, C. and Rollnick, S. (2008) 'How do child and family social workers talk to parents about child welfare concerns?' *Child Abuse Review 17*, 1, 23–35.

Frank, J. (1995) *Couldn't Care More: A Study of Young Carers and Their Needs.* London: The Children's Society.

Fraser, C., James, E. L., Anderson, K., Lloyd, D. and Judd, F. (2006) 'Interventions programmes for children of parents with a mental illness: A critical review.' *International Journal of Mental Health Promotion 8*, 1.

Fuller, R., Hallett, C., Murray, C. and Punch, S. (2000) *Young People and Welfare: Negotiating Pathways.* Stirling: University of Stirling, ESRC.

Galvani, S. (2010) *Grasping the Nettle: Alcohol and Domestic Violence* (revised ed.). London: University of Bedfordshire/Alcohol Concern.

Galvani, S. and Forrester, D. (2009) *Substance Use: Teaching the Basics: Learning and Teaching Guide.* Southampton: University of Bedfordshire, Higher Education Academy Subject Centre for Social Policy and Social Work (SWAP).

Galvani, S. and Livingstone, W. (2012) *Mental Health and Substance Use: Essential Information for Social Workers: A BASW Pocket Guide.* Birmingham: BASW.

Ghate, D., Shaw, C. and Hazel, N. (2000) *How Family Centres are Working with Fathers.* York: Joseph Rowntree Foundation.

Gopfert, M., Webster, J. and Seeman, M. (eds) (2004) *Parental Psychiatric Disorder: Distressed Parents and their Families.* Cambridge: Cambridge University Press.

Gorin, S. (2004) *Understanding What Children Say: Children's Experiences of Domestic Violence, Parental Substance Misuse and Parental Health Problems.* London: National Children's Bureau.

Gould, N. (2006) *Mental Health and Child Poverty.* York: Joseph Rowntree Foundation and University of Bath.

Greene, R., Pugh, R. and Roberts, D. (2008) *Black and Minority Ethnic Parents with Mental Health Problems and their Children.* Research Briefing 29. London: SCIE.

Grotberg, E (1997) *A guide to Promoting Resilience in Children: strengthening the human spirit.* Hague, Holland: Bernard van Leer Foundation.

Gruer, L. and Ainsworth, T. (2003) *Hidden Harm: Responding to the Needs of Children of Problem Drug Users. The Report of an Inquiry by the Advisory Council on the Misuse of Drugs.* London: Home Office.

Hamer, M. (2005) *Preventing Breakdown: A Manual for Those Working with Families and the Individuals Within Them.* Lyme Regis: Russell House Publishing.

Hamilton, C. and Collins, J. (1981) 'The Role of Alcohol in Wife Beating and Child Abuse: A Review of the Literature.' In J. Collins (ed.) *Drinking and Crime.* New York: Guilford Press.

Harbin, F. and Murphy, M. (eds) (2000) *Substance Misuse and Child Care: How to Understand, Assist and Intervene when Drugs Affect Parenting.* Lyme Regis: Russell House Publishing.

Hart, D. and Powell, J. (2006) *Adult Drug Problems, Children's Needs: Assessing the Impact of Parental Drug Use – A Toolkit for Practitioners.* London: National Children's Bureau.

Hawkins, A. J. and Dollahite, D. C. (eds) (1997) *Generative Fathering: Beyond Deficit Perspectives.* Thousand Oaks, CA: Sage.

Health Committee (2013) *Post Legislative Scrutiny of the Mental Health Act 2007.* London: The Stationery Office. Available at www.publications.parliament.uk/pa/cm201314/cmselect/cmhealth/584/584.pdf, accessed on 10 October 2015.

Hepburn M (2007) 'Drug use in pregnancy' in I.A. Greer, C. Nelson Pierc, Walter (eds) *Maternal Medicine: medical problems in pregnancy*. Philadelphia: L Health Sciences.

Hester, M., Pearson, C. and Harwin, N. (2003) 'Making an Impact: Children a. Domestic Violence – A Reader.' In B. Kroll and A. Taylor *Parental Substance Misuse and Child Welfare*. London: Jessica Kingsley Publishers.

X Hinshaw, S. (2005) 'The stigmatization of mental illness in children and parents: Developmental issues, family concerns, and research needs.' *Journal of Child Psychology and Psychiatry 46*, 7, 714–734.

HM Government (2006) *Common Assessment Framework guides*. London: HM Government.

HM Government (2008) *Drugs: Protecting Families and Communities. The 2008 Drug Strategy*. London: HM Government.

HM Government (2010) *Reducing Demand, Restricting Supply, Building Recovery: Supporting People to Live a Drug Free Life*. London: HM Government.

HM Government (2011) *Early Intervention: The Next Steps*. London: HM Government.

HM Government (2015) *Working Together to Safeguard Children: A Guide to Inter-agency Working to Safeguard and Promote the Welfare of Children*. London: HM Government.

Holland, S. (2004) *Child and Family Assessment in Social Work Practice*. London: Sage.

Hollows, A. (2003) 'Making Professional Judgements in the Framework for the Assessment of Children in Need and Their Families.' In M. C. Calder and S. Hackett (eds) *Assessment in Childcare: Using and Developing Frameworks for Practice*. Lyme Regis: Russell House Publishing.

Home Office, Department of Health and Department for Education (1995) *Tackling Drugs Together: A Strategy for England 1995–1998* (Cm 2846). London: HMSO.

Horwarth, J. (ed.) (2001) *The Child's World: Assessing Children in Need – World Training and Development Pack*. London: NSPCC.

Houmoller, K., Bernays, S., Wilson, S. and Rhodes, T. (2011) *Juggling Harms: Coping with Parental Substance Misuse*. London: School of Hygiene and Tropical Medicine.

ICAP (International Centre for Alcohol Policies) (2011) *The ICAP Blue Book – Practice Guides for Alcohol Policy and Prevention Approaches. Module 22: Alcohol and the Work Place*. Washington, DC: International Centre for Alcohol Policies.

X Jack, G. (1997) 'An ecological approach to social work with children and families.' *Child and Family Social Work 2*, 109–120.

Jack, G. and Gill, O. (2003) *The Missing Side of the Triangle: Assessing the Importance of Family and Environmental Factors in the Lives of Children*. Barkingside: Barnardo's.

Jones, A., Jeyasingham, D., and Rajaasooriya, S. (2002) *Invisible families: The strengths ofblack families in which young people have caring responsibilities*. Bristol: The Policy Press.

Kearney, P., Levin, E. and Rosen, G. (2003a) *Alcohol, Drug and Mental Health Problems: Working with Families* (SCIE Report 2). London: SCIE.

Kearney, P., Levin, E., Rosen, G. and Sainsbury, M. (2003b) *Families that have Alcohol and Mental Health Problems: A Template for Partnership Working* (SCIE Resource Guide 1). London: SCIE.

Kirkman, E. and Melrose, K. (2014) *Clinical Judgement and Decision-Making in Children's Social Work: An Analysis of the 'Front Door' System: Research Report*. London: Department for Education.

Kroll, B. and Taylor, A. (2003) *Parental Substance Misuse and Child Welfare*. London: Jessica Kingsley Publishers.

Kroll, B. and Taylor, A. (2008) *Interventions for Children and Families where there is Parental Drug Misuse.* Exeter: ARTEC Enterprises Ltd.

Kurtz, Z., Stapelkamp, C., Taylor, E., Malek, M. and Street, C. (2005) *Minority Voices: A Guide to Good Practice in Planning and Providing Services for the Mental Health of Black and Minority Ethnic Young People.* London: Young Minds.

Lam, C.B., McHale, S.M., & Crouter, M. (2012). Parent–child shared time from middle childhood to late adolescence: developmental course and adjustment correlates. *Child Development, 83,* 6, 2089–2103.

Lavis, P. (2014) *Better Health Briefing: The Importance of Promoting Mental Health in Children and Young People from Black and Minority Ethnic Communities.* A Race Equality Foundation Briefing Paper. London: Children and Young People's Mental Health Coalition, Race Equality Foundation.

Laybourn, A., Brown, J. and Hill, M. (1996) *Hurting on the Inside: Children's Experience of Parental Alcohol Misuse.* Aldershot: Avebury.

Leese, M., Thornicroft, G., Shaw, J., Thomas, S., *et al.* (2006) 'Ethnic differences among patients in high-security psychiatric hospitals in England.' *British Journal of Psychiatry 188,* 380–385.

Link, B. G., Struening, E. L., Rahav, M., Phelan, J. C. and Nuttbrock, L. (1997) 'On stigma and its consequences: Evidence from a longitudinal study of men with dual diagnoses of mental illness and substance abuse.' *Journal of Health and Social Behaviour 38,* 177–190.

Link, B.G., Phelan, J.C., Bresnahan, M., Stueve, A. and Pescosolido, B.A. (1999). 'Public conception of mental illness: Labels, causes, dangerousness, and social distance', *American Journal of Public Health.*

Lyall, J. (2006) 'The struggle for 'cultural competence.' *The Guardian,* 12 April.

Malek, M. (2011) *Enjoy, Achieve and be Healthy: The Mental Health of Black and Minority Ethnic Children and Young People.* London: Afiya Trust.

Manning, V., Best, D, Faulkner, N. and Titherington, E. (2009) 'New estimates of the number of children living with substance misusing parents: results from the UK National Household Surveys.' *BMC Public Health 9,* 377.

Martins, C. (2013) *Strategic Prompt: Parental Substance Misuse.* Totnes: Research in Practice.

McCarthy, T. and Galvani, S. (2010) *Alcohol and other Drugs – Essential Information for Social Workers. A BASW Pocket Guide.* Luton: University of Bedfordshire.

McCarthy, T. and Galvani, S. (2012) *Children, Families and Alcohol Use: Essential Information for Social Workers. A BASW Pocket Guide.* Birmingham: BASW.

McCracken, D. G. (1988) *The Long Interview.* Beverly Hills, CA: Sage.

Meltzer, H., Gill, B. and Petticrew, M. (1995) *OPCS Surveys of Psychiatric Morbidity in Great Britain. Report No 1. The Prevalence of Psychiatric Morbidity Among Adults Aged 16-64 Living in Private Households in Great Britain.* London: HMSO.

Melzer, D. (2003) 'Inequalities in Mental Health: A Systematic Review. The Research Findings Register, Summary no. 1063.' In Family Welfare Association (2008) *Families Affected by Parental Mental Health Difficulties.* London: Family Welfare Association.

Miller, N. S. (ed.) (1994) *Treating Coexisting Psychiatric and Addictive Disorders.* Center City, MN: Hazelden.

Miller, W. R. and Rollnick, S. (2002) *Motivational Interviewing: Preparing People for Change.* New York: Guilford Press.

Miller, W. R. and Rollnick, S. (2012) *Motivational Interviewing: Helping People Change* (3rd edition). New York: Guilford Press.

Morris, J. and Wates, M. (2006) *Supporting Disabled Parents and Parents with Additional Support Needs*. Knowledge Review 11. London: SCIE.

Mullender, A., Hague, G., Imam, U., Kelly, L., Malos, E. and Regan, L. (2002) *Children's Perspectives on Domestic Violence*. London: Sage.

Newman, T. and Blackburn, S. (2002) *Transitions in the Lives of Children and Young People: Resilience Factors* (Interchange 78). Edinburgh: Scottish Executive.

NHS England and NHS Improving Quality (2014) *Commitment for Carers: Report of the Findings and Outcomes*. London: NHS Improving Quality.

NSPCC (2000) *The Child's World: Assessing Children in Need*. London: NSPCC.

NSPCC Information Service (2015) *Hidden Men: Learning from Case Reviews: Summary of Risk Factors and Learning for Improved Practice Around 'Hidden' Men*. London: NSPCC Information Service.

NTA (National Treatment Agency) (2012) *Parents with Drug Problems: How Treatment Helps Families*. London: National Treatment Agency.

Ofsted (2011) *Learning Lessons from Serious Case Reviews 2009–2010*. London: Ofsted.

Ofsted (2014) *An Overview of Inspection Findings from OFSTED, CQC, HMIC*. London: Ofsted.

Olsen, R. and Wates, M. (2003) *Disabled Parents: Examining Research Assumptions*. Totnes: Research in Practice.

Parrott, L., Jacobs, G. and Roberts, D. (2008) *Stress and Resilience Factors in Parents with Mental health Problems and their Children*. Research Briefing 23. London: SCIE.

Patel, N. (ed.) (2000) *Clinical Psychology, Race, and Culture: A Training Manual*. Leicester: British Psychological Society.

Peisah, C., Brodaty, H., Luscome, G. and Anstey, K. J. (2004) 'Children of a cohort of depressed parents 25 years later: Psychopathology and relationships.' *Journal of Affective Disorders 82*, 3, 385–394.

Phillips, E. (ed.) (2004) *Children Exposed to Parental Substance Misuse: Implications for Family Placement*. London: BAAF.

Pitman, E. (1997) *Simplifying Mental Illness plus Life Enhancement Skills (SMILES)*. Information Sheet.

Powers, R. (1986) 'Aggression and Violence in the Family.' In A. Campbell and J. Gibbs *Violent Transactions*. Oxford: Basil Blackwell.

Prime Minister's Strategy Unit (2003) *Alcohol Harm Reduction Project: Interim Analytical Report*. London: Cabinet Office.

Prochaska, J. O., Norcross, J. C. and Diclemente, C. C. (1994) *Changing for Good: The Revolutionary Program that Explains the Six Stages of Change and Teaches You How to Free Yourself from Bad Habits*. New York: William Morrow and Co.

Raynes, B. (2003) 'A Stepwise Process of Assessment' in Calder, M. C. and Hackett, S. (eds) *Assessment in child care: Using and developing frameworks for practice. Second edition*. Dorset: Russell House Publishing.

Rayns, G., Dawe, S. and Cuthbert, C. (2013) *All Babies Count: Spotlight on Drugs and Alcohol*. London: NSPCC.

Roberts, A. R. (1990) *Crisis Intervention Handbook: Assessment, Treatment and Research*. Belmont CA: Wadsworth.

Roberts, A. (2005) *Crisis Intervention Handbook: Assessment, Treatment and Research* (3rd ed.). Oxford: OUP.

Rogers, C. (1962) *On Becoming a Person: A Therapist's View Of Psychotherapy*. London: Constable.

Roskill, C., Featherstone, B., Ashley, C. and Haresnape, S. (2008) *Fathers Matter Volume 2: Further Findings on Fathers and their Involvement with Social Care Service.* London: Family Rights Group.

Rutter, M. (1993) 'Resilience: Some conceptual considerations.' *Journal of Adolescent Health 14*, 626–631.

Rutter, M. (1999) 'Resilience concepts and findings: Implications for family therapy.' *Journal of Family Therapy 21*, 119–144.

Ryan, M. (2000) *Working with Fathers.* Abingdon: Radcliffe Medical Press.

Sartorius, N. (1998) 'Stigma: What can psychiatrists do about it?' *Lancet 352*, 1058–1059.

SCIE (Social Care Institute for Excellence) (2011) *Think Child, Think Parent, Think Family: A Guide to Parental Mental Health and Child Welfare – Summary.* London: Social Care Institute for Excellence. Available at: www.scie.org.uk/publications/guides/guide30/summary.asp, accessed on 14 October 2015.

SCIE (Social Care Institute for Excellence) (2012) *Think Child, Think Parent, Think Family: Putting it into Practice – At a Glance Briefing 55.* London: Social Care Institute for Excellence.

Scott, D. (1998) 'A qualitative study of social work assessment in cases of alleged child abuse.' *British Journal of Social Work 28*, 1, 73–88.

Sheldon, B. (1987) 'The Psychology of Incompetence.' In L. Blom-Cooper (ed.) *After Beckford: Essays on Themes Connected with the Case of Jasmine Beckford.* London: Royal Holloway and Bedford New College.

Social Exclusion Unit (2004) *Mental Health and Social Exclusion.* London: Office of the Deputy Prime Minister.

Somers, V. (2006) '*Schizophrenia: the impact of parental illness on children.*' *British Journal of Social Work 37*, 8, 1319–1334.

Spector, A. (2006) 'Fatherhood and depression: A review of risks, effects and clinical application.' *Issues in Mental Health Nursing 27*, 8, 867–883.

Taylor, A. (2013) *The Impact of Parental Substance Misuse on Child Development. Frontline Briefing.* Totnes: Research in Practice.

Templeton, L., Zohhadi, S., Galvani, S. and Velleman, R. (2006) *Looking Beyond Risk. Parental Substance Misuse: Scoping Study.* Edinburgh: Mental Health Research and Development Unit (University of Bath, Avon and Wiltshire Mental Health Partnership NHS Trust and University of Birmingham) Scottish Executive Substance Misuse Research Programme.

Thornicroft, G. (2006) *Actions Speak Louder… Tackling Discrimination Against People with Mental Illness.* London: Mental Health Foundation.

Time to Change (2008) *Stigma Shout Survey: Service User and Carer Experiences of Stigma and Discrimination.* Available at: www.time-to-change.org.uk/sites/default/files/Stigma%20Shout.pdf, accessed on 14 October 2015.

Treasure, J. (2004) 'Motivational interviewing.' *Advances in Psychiatric Treatment 10*, 331–337.

Tunnard, J. (2002a) *Parental Drug Misuse: A Review of Impact and Intervention Studies.* Totnes: Research in Practice.

Tunnard, J. (2002b) *Parental Problem Drinking and its Impact on Children.* Totnes: Research in Practice.

Tunnard, J. (2004) *Parental Mental Health Problems: Messages from Research, Policy and Practice.* Totnes: Research in Practice.

Turnell, A. and Edwards, S. (1999) *Signs of Safety: A Solution and Safety-orientated Approach to Child Protection.* New York: WW Norton and Co.

Turning Point (2006) *Bottling It Up: The Effects of Alcohol Misuse on Children, Parents and Families.* London: Turning Point.

Turning Point (2007) *Dual Diagnosis Good Practice Handbook.* London: Turning Point.

UKDPC (2010a) *Drugs and Diversity: Ethnic Minority Groups.* London: UKDPC.

UKDPC (2010b) *Getting Serious About Stigma: The Problem with Stigmatising Drug Users.* London: UKDPC.

Velleman, R. (1993) *Alcohol and the Family.* London: Institute of Alcohol Studies.

Velleman, R. (2004) 'Alcohol and Drug Problems in Parents: An Overview of the Impact on Children and Implications for Practice.' In M. Gopfert, J. Webster and M. Seeman (eds) *Parental Psychiatric Disorder: Distressed Parents and their Families.* Cambridge: Cambridge University Press.

Velleman, R. and Orford, J. (1993) 'The importance of family discord in explaining childhood problems.' *Addiction Research 1,* 1, 36–57.

Velleman, R. and Orford, J. (1999) *Risk and Resilience: Adults who were the Children of Problem Drinkers.* Reading: Harwood.

Wahl, O. F. (1995) *Media Madness: Public Images of Mental Illness.* New Brunswick, NJ: Rutgers University Press.

World Health Organization (1992) *The ICD10 Classification of Mental and Behavioural Disorders: Clinical Descriptions and Diagnostic Guidelines.* Geneva: WHO.

Further reading

Bowyer, S., Harnett, P. and Dawe, S. (2013) *Assessing Parents' Capacity to Change.* Frontline briefing, Research in Practice. Dartington: Research in Practice.

Brandon, M., Bailey, S., Belderson, P. and Larsson, B. (2013) *Neglect and Serious Case Reviews.* London: University of East Anglia/NSPCC.

Department for Education (2011) *Family and Friends Care: Statutory Guidance for Local Authorities.* London: Department for Education.

Department for Education and Skills (2005) *Statutory Guidance on the Roles and Responsibilities of the Director of Children's Services and Lead Member for Children's Services.* London: Department for Education and Skills.

Harwin, J., Ryan, M., Tunnard, J., Pokhrel, S., *et al.* (2011) *The Family Drug and Alcohol Court (FDAC) Evaluation Project Final Reports.* London: Brunel University.

NSPCC (2013) *Learning from Case Reviews Involving Parental Substance Misuse.* London: NSPCC.

NSPCC (2013) *Learning from Case Reviews Where Domestic Abuse Was a Key Factor.* London: NSPCC.

Turney, D. (2014) *Analysis and Critical Thinking in Assessment: Literature Review* (Second edition). Dartington: Research in Practice.

Wates, M. (2002) *Supporting Disabled Adults in their Parenting Role.* York: Joseph Rowntree Foundation.

Appendix
Building resilience in families under stress – Policy annex update

Zoe Renton and Keith Clements, April 2015

This appendix covers the following relevant areas of policy and law:

- cross-cutting service provision
- children's and adult social care
- health services
- welfare reform
- mental health
- drugs and alcohol
- families and parenting
- disability.

1. Cross-cutting service provision
Human Rights Act 1998

The government incorporated the European Convention on Human Rights into UK law in 1998, creating the Human Rights Act. The most relevant articles are:

- Article 3, which prohibits inhuman and degrading treatment
- Article 8, which guarantees the right to respect for private and family life
- Article 14, prohibiting discrimination in the enjoyment of Convention rights.

Article 8 is of particular significance, since it prohibits any arbitrary interference with the right to a private and family life. For example, case law stipulates that even though a child may be taken into care for his or her protection, this does not allow for the relationship between the child and birth parent to be terminated unless this is in the best interests of the child.

Article 3 stipulates that protection rights are absolute, so children should be protected from all forms of inhuman and degrading treatment. What is less clear, however, is the demarcation line under Article 3 that requires that action be taken by social services or other state agencies to protect that child.

UN Convention on the Rights of the Child (UNCRC)

The UK government ratified the CRC in 1991. While the government formerly reserved the right to insist on the primacy of UK immigration law over Convention rights, this reservation was withdrawn in 2008. The CRC has not been incorporated into UK law and, unlike the European Convention on Human Rights, has no court system attached to ensure that it is understood and implemented.

The most relevant articles are:

- Article 3 – best interests of a child (in all actions, the best interests of the child shall be a primary consideration)
- Article 5 – parental guidance (which deals with the responsibilities, rights and duties of parents for their child)
- Article 9 – separation from parents (which ensures that a child may not be separated from his or her parents against their will, unless it is necessary to protect the child from harm or in cases involving parental separation that specify a child's place of residence)
- Article 19 – protection from abuse and neglect.

Equality Act 2010

The Equality Act 2010 aims to consolidate all previous anti-discrimination and equality legislation, as well as strengthening protection from discrimination, harassment or victimisation in relation to age, disability, gender, race, religion or belief, sexuality, gender reassignment, marriage and civil partnership and pregnancy and maternity. It also introduces a new 'public sector equality duty', requiring all public bodies to eliminate unlawful discrimination, harassment or victimisation, and promote equality of opportunity and good relations. The Equality and Human Rights Commission (EHRC) has duties and powers under the Equality Act 2006 to enforce anti-discriminatory legislation (including the 2010 act) and promote a culture of respect for human rights.

Children's services

The Children Act 2004 provides a legislative framework for partnership working across agencies to promote children's well-being. This framework includes:

- a reciprocal duty on a list of local partners (including local authorities, health services, the police and probation, schools and colleges and youth offending teams) to cooperate to improve the well-being of children (section 10)
- a definition of child well-being: physical and mental health and emotional well-being; protection from harm and neglect; access to education, training and recreation; making a contribution to society; and social and economic well-being (section 10)
- a duty on partners to safeguard and promote the welfare of children (section 11)
- every local authority having to appoint a Director of Children's Services and a named councillor or 'lead member' with responsibility for children's services (sections 18 and 19)
- the requirement that each local area have a Local Safeguarding Children Board (section 13).

Related cross-government guidance includes:

- *Working Together to Safeguard Children: A Guide to Inter-agency Working to Safeguard and Promote the Welfare of Children* (HM Government 2015a), statutory guidance www.gov.uk/government/publications/working-together-to-safeguard-children--2
- *Information Sharing: Guidance for Practitioners and Managers* (HM Government 2008), department advice. www.gov.uk/government/publications/information-sharing-for-practitioners-and-managers.

Joint and integrated inspections

Ofsted, along with its counterparts in health, probation, policing and prisons, has powers to undertake joint inspections. The inspectorates use these powers to carry out a programme of targeted inspections to evaluate how local agencies work together to protect children, focused on specific areas of concern. A more formal system of regular, integrated inspections was piloted and consulted on in 2014, but following this it was decided that these proposals would not be taken forward.[1]

---

1   www.gov.uk/government/consultations/integrated-inspections-of-services-for-children-in-need-of-help-and-protection-children-looked-after-care-leavers-joint-inspection-of-the-local-s

2. Children's and adult social care

Children Act 1989

The Children Act 1989 is the major child-centred piece of social welfare legislation. Section 1 contains the heart of the Act: the welfare of the child should be the core consideration whenever a court is required to make a decision regarding the upbringing of a child, or administration of a child's property. The Act introduces the concept of parental responsibility – given automatically to birth mothers and married fathers, and upon application to an unmarried father – which in law refers to 'the rights, duties, powers, responsibilities and authority which by law a parent of a child has in relation to the child and his property'. Parents who separate may still have parental responsibility and are expected to maintain some involvement in their child's life. When considering the welfare of a child, the court uses the welfare checklist as a framework within which to make its decision. The checklist comprises:

- the ascertainable wishes and feelings of the child concerned (considered in the light of his age and understanding)
- his physical, emotional and educational needs
- the likely effect on him of any change in his circumstances
- his age, sex, background and any characteristics of his which the court considers relevant
- any harm that he has suffered or is at risk of suffering
- how capable each of his parents, and any other person in relation to whom the court considers the question to be relevant, is of meeting his needs
- the range of powers available to the court.

Part III of the Act deals with local authority duties. Section 17 deals with the provision of services for children in need. A child is 'in need' if: he or she is unlikely to achieve or maintain, or to have the opportunity of achieving or maintaining, a reasonable standard of health or development without the provision of services; or the child's health or development is likely to be significantly impaired, or further impaired, without the provision of such services; or the child is disabled. Children who are suffering or at risk of suffering 'significant harm' may be taken into the care of the local authority. The harm must be attributable to the care given to the child or the child being beyond parental control.

The Children and Families Act 2014 includes amendments to the 1989 Act setting out the duties of local authorities to young carers, requiring that they carry out an assessment of a young carer's needs including assessing whether the child should continue to provide care (Sections 17 ZA-ZC in the Children Act 1989). The needs of young carers are also considered under the Care Act 2014 and associated guidance.

Child protection

In June 2010, the government commissioned Professor Eileen Munro to conduct a review of the child protection system. Her final report (Department for Education 2011a) was published in May 2011, followed by the government's response in July of the same year (Department for Education 2011b). Munro emphasised the need to 'move from a compliance to a learning culture', allowing freedom for social workers to use their professional judgement (Department for Education 2011a, p.62). Her recommendations included measures to: remove unhelpful targets, IT systems and guidelines; secure early help for families who do not meet the criteria for social care services to prevent problems escalating; and keep experienced social workers on the front line.

Since the Munro review, the Government published revised versions of *Working Together to Safeguard Children* statutory guidance, the latest in March 2015 (HM Government 2015a), along with versions for children and young people. The guidance emphasises two key principles: that safeguarding is everyone's responsibility – including teachers, GPs, nurses, midwives, health visitors, early years professionals, youth workers, police, accident and emergency staff, paediatricians, voluntary and community workers and social workers; and that services should be based on the needs and views of children. It highlights the role of all professionals, including those supporting adults with children, to identify emerging problems and share information to secure early help for children and families that need it. In addition, the government published *Information Sharing: Advice for Practitioners Providing Safeguarding Services to Children, Young People, Parents and Carers* (Department for Education 2015a) to help frontline practitioners working in child or adult services make decisions about sharing personal information. In addition, in 2013 the then NHS Commissioning Board (now NHS England) published *Safeguarding Vulnerable People in the Reformed NHS: Accountability and Assurance Framework* (NHS Commissioning Board 2015), seeking to provide clarity about the safeguarding responsibilities of health service leaders, commissioners, providers and regulators.

Care Act 2014

Part 1 of the Care Act 2014 sets out the core legal duties and powers relating to adult social care. Most of the Act came into force in April 2015, with some additional provisions due to be implemented from April 2016.

Top-tier local authorities have duties to assess and meet the needs of adults in need of care and support and their carers. This includes an overarching duty to promote the well-being of these individuals, which includes reference to their physical and mental health and emotional well-being and their domestic, family and personal relationships, among other considerations.

The eligibility threshold for adults with care and support needs is set out in the Care and Support (Eligibility Criteria) Regulations 2014 (the 'Eligibility Regulations'). The threshold is based on identifying how a person's needs affect their ability to achieve relevant outcomes and how this impacts on their well-being. In considering whether an adult with care and support needs has eligible needs, local authorities must consider whether:

- the adult's needs arise from or are related to a physical or mental impairment or illness (this includes substance misuse)
- as a result of the adult's needs the adult is unable to achieve two or more of the specified outcomes (these include carrying out any caring responsibilities they have for a child, developing and maintaining family or other personal relationships and maintaining a habitable home environment)
- as a consequence of being unable to achieve these outcomes there is, or there is likely to be, a significant impact on the adult's well-being.

Local authorities are allowed to charge for care and support services for adults, subject to the principle that people are only charged what they can afford to pay and a number of other requirements set out in regulations.

Part 1 of the Care Act and related regulations are complemented and explained in more detail by the *Care and Support Statutory Guidance* (Department of Health 2014a). The guidance makes clear that children should not undertake inappropriate or excessive caring roles that may have an impact on their development. It also reminds local authorities that where a young carer is identified, the local authority must undertake a young carer's assessment under Part 3 of the Children Act 1989.

As well as assessing and meeting existing needs, the Act places duties on local authorities to take steps to prevent, delay and reduce needs for care and support in its area. They must provide information to individuals about what can be done in this regard.

While main duties in the Act only apply for those aged over 18, it contains a number of provisions on the transition for children's to adults' services including:

- a duty to assess before their 18th birthday, the needs of a young person caring for an adult, which, in cases where a young person is experiencing or at risk of abuse and neglect, applies regardless of whether the young person consents to this
- a duty to assess before their 18th birthday, the needs of a young person likely to have care and support needs as an adult
- a duty to assess before their child's 18th birthday, the needs of a parent caring for a child with care and support needs, and a power to meet those needs
- a number of provisions regarding continuity of care across various legal frameworks.

3. Health services

The current structure and legal framework of the NHS in England was established by the Health and Social Care Act 2012, and the amendments this Act made to existing legislation such as the National Health Service Act 2006 and the Local Government and Public Involvement in Health Act 2007.

In total, 211 Clinical Commissioning Groups (CCGs) carry out local commissioning of most NHS services to meet the physical and mental health needs of their populations. CCGs are led by groups of GP practices, but also include other medical professionals and lay members on their governing bodies.

NHS England (referred to in law as the NHS Commissioning Board) oversees the NHS and commissions NHS services that cannot be commissioned by CCGs. These include specialist services such as inpatient CAMHS and all health and public health services for the prison population. It allocates funding to CCGs and supports and assures their work. Most of NHS England's work is carried out through its 27 area teams.

Local authorities are responsible for promoting and protecting the health of their local areas and are required to commission particular services as part of doing this. From October 2015, this includes responsibility for commissioning the Family Nurse Partnership programme and the Healthy Child Programme 0–5, including health visiting services, with key aspects of the programme set out as requirements in regulations. Local authorities' public health role also includes responsibility for the Healthy Child Programme 5–19, led by school nurses, and substance misuse services for people of all ages, although no specific model or level of service is required by law. Local authorities receive a ring-fenced Public Health Grant to carry out this role and employ Directors of Public Health, who lead the work.

Health and well-being boards are cross agency fora that plan local health, public health and social care services by producing a Joint Strategic Needs Assessment and Health and Wellbeing Strategy. Statutory guidance on this process states that Health and Wellbeing Boards will need to consider 'how needs may be harder to meet for those in disadvantaged areas or vulnerable groups who experience inequalities', with troubled families being listed as one example of such a group (Department of Health 2013, p.8).

Most agencies involved in the health service have similar duties to have regard to the need to reduce inequalities in access to health services and in health outcomes.

4. Welfare reform

The Welfare Reform Act 2012, following the publication of a welfare reform white paper (Department for Work and Pensions 2010), introduced a programme of changes to the welfare system. Existing work-related benefits – including Income Support (for those on low incomes), Employment and Support Allowance (for those who are unable to work because of illness or disability), Jobseeker's Allowance, Housing Benefit, Child Tax Credit and Working Tax Credit – are to be integrated into a single Universal Credit (UC). The single, basic UC payment, providing for basic living costs, will be augmented by additional amounts for certain circumstances, including: disability; caring responsibilities; housing costs; number of children; and childcare. There will be a phased approach to the introduction of UC starting in 2015, although there has been limited roll-out since April 2013. At the time of writing, the government is aiming for all claimants to be on UC by the end of 2017.

In 2013, also under the Welfare Reform Act 2012, the government introduced a cap on the amount of benefits households can receive for those in receipt of UC or Housing Benefit. Those receiving Disability Living Allowance, war widows and working families will be exempt from the cap. Some recipients now face an increasing level of conditionality. Recipients of UC are subject to a 'claimant commitment', outlining the work-related requirements expected of them, with tougher sanctions if these are not met.

5. Mental health
Mental Health Act 1983 and the Code of Practice

The Mental Health Act 1983 – amended by the Mental Health Act 2007 – provides a framework for compulsory admissions to hospital, treatment in the community and provisions for the care of inpatients and aftercare. It sets out the following broad principles: respect and consideration of individual qualities; needs taken fully into account; treatment or care to be in the least controlled and segregated facilities practicable; and self-determination of service users to be supported as far as possible. Discharge from orders are to take place as soon as appropriate. Key sections are:

- Section 2 – compulsory admission for assessment (up to 28 days)
- Section 3 – compulsory admission for treatment (up to six months renewable for a further six months, then annually)
- Section 4 – compulsory admission in an emergency (where there is an urgent need for admission for assessment and compliance with procedure under Section 2 could cause undesirable delay); this lasts up to 72 hours and is for use in genuine emergencies. This is closely regulated by the Mental Health Act Commission and includes holding powers for doctors and nurses – Section 5(2) and 5(4)
- Section 37 – a hospital order can be made where someone who would normally receive a prison sentence is convicted of an offence (a 'treatability' test applies)
- Section 117 – aftercare: a duty on local authorities in relation to people who have been admitted under sections 3, 37, 45(a), 47 or 48 of the Act to provide aftercare on discharge
- Section 136 – police powers: where police can remove someone to a place of safety for up to 72 hours, the aim being to secure competent and speedy assessment by a doctor and Approved Social Worker (ASW) of the person. Local areas should have clear policies regarding the use of this.

A statutory Code of Practice contains a number of directions regarding patients who are parents, including regarding sharing information with their children and visiting rights (Department of Health 2015).

Mental health policy

The 2011 mental health strategy, *No Health Without Mental Health* (HM Government 2011a), sets out priorities for promoting good mental health among all age groups. It highlights the importance of intervening early to address mental health problems, and in particular the damaging effect of a parent's poor mental health on their children. There is also an emphasis on: promoting 'positive parenting' as a means of preventing mental health problems among children and young people; parental anxiety and depression in the postnatal period and early years; and the importance of addressing the needs of children of a parent with mental health problems to prevent them from taking on inappropriate caring roles.

Closing the Gap (Department of Health 2014b), published in January 2014, aims to bridge the gap between the long-term ambitions set out in the strategy and shorter term action. Priorities and commitments include: waiting time limits for mental health services; tackling inequalities around access to mental health services; better supporting of and involving carers; giving adults the right to make choices about their care; and support for employers and schools to address mental health. There is also a commitment to improve support for new mothers to minimise the impacts of postnatal depression by updating and expanding training for midwives and health visitors.

The Children and Young People's Mental Health and Wellbeing Taskforce was established in September 2014 to consider ways to make it easier for children, young people, parents and carers to access help and support when needed and to improve how children and young people's mental health services are organised, commissioned and provided. Its report, *Future in Mind*, published in March 2015, sets out wide-ranging proposals for reform (Department of Health and NHS England 2015). The aspirations it sets out include improving access for parents to evidence-based programmes of intervention and support to strengthen attachment between parent and child and a better offer for the most vulnerable children and young people, making it easier for them to access the support that they need when and where they need it.

Practice resources from NICE and SCIE

The Social Care Institute for Excellence (SCIE) has developed a range of resources on parental mental health and child welfare (including dual diagnosis) and provides good practice examples.[2]

The National Institute for Health and Care Excellence (NICE) has published a range of practice guidance on topics such as promoting the social and emotional well-being of children in the early years, primary and secondary education, alcohol use disorders and drug misuse.[3]

---

2 www.scie.org.uk/atoz

3 www.nice.org.uk/guidance

6. Drugs and alcohol

Following reforms to the health and social care system, since April 2013 local authorities have been responsible for drug and alcohol information, support and treatment services, supported by Public Health England. Public Health England has taken over the functions of the former National Treatment Agency for Substance Misuse.

Drug Strategy 2010

In December 2010, the coalition government published a revised drug strategy (HM Government 2010), progress on which is reported in annual reviews (for the latest review, see HM Government 2015b). It addresses drug and alcohol dependency and highlights the association between mental illness and drug and alcohol dependence. There is an emphasis on preventing problems from arising, referring to government policies relating to Sure Start Children's Centres and interventions for families with multiple problems. Stating that children are sometimes 'invisible' to drug and alcohol services working with parents, the strategy stresses that children and adult services should work together to protect children in accordance with *Working Together to Safeguard Children* statutory guidance (see earlier), and encourages those working with children and families affected by substance misuse to undertake appropriate training. It encourages drug and alcohol, family and children's services to develop protocols for working together to respond to safeguarding concerns and support parents through treatment and in caring for their children, referring to National Treatment Agency guidelines. The strategy states that drug and alcohol services should be represented on Local Safeguarding Children Boards.

Alcohol Strategy 2012

The coalition government's alcohol strategy (HM Government 2012) outlines action to: reduce the availability of cheap alcohol; give local agencies powers and tools to tackle alcohol-related problems and reduce health inequalities; and support individuals to drink responsibly. It recognises that a third of adults in alcohol treatment are parents with childcare responsibilities, and refers to alcohol treatment and children's and family services working more closely together, including through Family Intervention Projects and the Troubled Families programme (see later). Referring to Foetal Alcohol Spectrum Disorder (FASD), it commits government to continued awareness raising around drinking during pregnancy and when trying to conceive. The guidance encourages NHS health professionals routinely to carry out alcohol screening and says that government expects all areas to implement the NICE guidance and quality standard on harmful drinking and alcohol dependence (National Institute for Health and Care Excellence 2011).

Hidden Harm

In 2003, the Advisory Council on the Misuse of Drugs published research and policy recommendations on responding to the needs of children of problem drug users (Gruer and Ainsworth 2003). Its report, *Hidden Harm*, estimated that there were between

250,000 and 350,000 children of problem drug users in the UK. It notes that parental drug use can and does cause serious harm to children at every stage from conception to adulthood, and it recommends that reducing the harm to children from parental problem drug use should become a main objective of policy and practice. The principle of services working together is highlighted, as is the recognition that effective treatment of the parent can have major benefits for the child (see also Advisory Council on the Misuse of Drugs 2007, 2011).

Misuse of Drugs Act 1971

This Act categorises controlled drugs into three classes, with Class A drugs (that is, heroin, cocaine and ecstasy) considered to be the most harmful and Class C drugs less harmful. For Class A drugs, the maximum sentence for possession is currently seven years' imprisonment and an unlimited fine; for supply, it is life imprisonment and an unlimited fine. The possession of Class B drugs can lead to a maximum five years' imprisonment or a fine or both; for supply, 14 years' imprisonment, a fine or both. Drugs not covered by the Act include alcohol and solvents. However, the 1971 Act was amended in 2011, giving the government powers to introduce 'temporary class drug orders' to tackle manufacturers of 'legal highs' (amended by the Police Reform and Social Responsibility Act 2011).

Criminal justice and drugs and alcohol

Drug testing and treatment orders were introduced in the Crime and Disorder Act 1998; and were replaced through the Criminal Justice Act 2003 by drug rehabilitation requirements in 2005. These are community orders that may be imposed on drug-dependent offenders who may be susceptible to treatment in areas where the appropriate services are deemed to be available. If the offender refuses to comply with the order, they can be subject to either a maximum £5000 fine or a custodial sentence. The treatment provider – with treatment being either residential or non-residential – will act as the main supervisor of drug testing and the court may undertake periodic reviews, which must initially at least be attended by the offender. The Criminal Justice Act 2003 also introduced an alcohol treatment requirement, another community sentence that requires offenders to submit to treatment.

For adult offenders released from prison, the Offender Rehabilitation Act 2014 introduces a new licence condition that can require them to attend appointments designed to address their dependency on or propensity to misuse drugs.

Models of care for alcohol and drug misusers

In 2006, the Department of Health and NTA published a guide to the commissioning of alcohol services, which included a short chapter on assessment that covers parenting responsibilities, and refers concerned professionals to the Local Safeguarding Children Board and social services (NTA/Department of Health 2006). A similar document provides national guidance on the commissioning and provision of treatment for adult drug misusers (NTA/Department of Health/Home Office 2006). It sets out care pathways for parents or pregnant women known to be misusing drugs and advocates a harm reduction approach with service users' children and families. The functions of the NTA have been brought into Public Health England (PHE) and, according to the Drug Strategy Annual Review for 2014–15, PHE will be undertaking projects on the impact of parental alcohol use (HM Government 2015b).

Other useful resources

In 2007, the Department of Health (England), the Scottish Government, Welsh Assembly Government and Northern Ireland Executive published *Drug Misuse and Dependence: UK Guidelines on Clinical Management*. It has been agreed that these guidelines will be updated for early 2016.[4]

SCIE provides e-learning on parental substance misuse (2011). Its 2003 report, *Working with Families with Alcohol, Drug and Mental Health Problems*, provides advice on promoting integrated services to families.[5]

7. Families and parenting

Early years

Supporting Families in the Foundation Years (Department for Education/Department of Health 2011) brings together the government's policies around pregnancy up to the age of five, and describes the systems needed to make the government's vision for services for children, parents and families of this age group a reality.

The document emphasises the importance of parental health and well-being to children's development, highlighting issues such as mental health, drug and alcohol misuse and poor family relationships.

As well as outlining policies relating to early education and childcare, the document included commitments to support parents of young children. It confirmed the government's commitment to double the number of families (to 13,000) accessing the Family Nurse Partnership programme – a preventive programme, developed in the USA, providing intensive structured home visiting for young first-time mothers. This has since been extended to reach 16,000 young new mothers by 2015. The government also committed to recruiting a further 4200 health visitors by 2015. From 2012 to 2014, the Department for Education trialled the delivery of free parenting classes for mothers and fathers of children aged up to five in three local authority areas (the CANparent programme) to test the market for universal, stigma-free parenting classes.

---

4   www.gov.uk/government/consultations/drug-misuse-and-dependence-uk-guidelines-on-clinical-management

5   www.scie.org.uk/atoz

Early intervention

In June 2010, the coalition government commissioned Graham Allen MP to conduct a review into early intervention, including how to secure, deliver and fund effective prevention and early intervention services (HM Government 2011b). The government's response to Allen's review has centred on its policies for the early years (described above). In addition, in the *Spending Review 2010* (HM Treasury 2010), the government announced that local areas would receive an Early Intervention Grant (EIG), bringing together a range of funding streams for children, young people and families, including funding for family support, early years and youth services.

The EIG represented a cut in funding for these services and is not ring-fenced, and the level of funding has continued to fall. However, the government is encouraging local areas to use it to support a range of services, including targeted support for families with multiple problems and ensuring Children's Centres are accessible to all (but focusing support on the most vulnerable families).

The Troubled Families programme

In December 2010, the prime minister set out an ambition to, by 2015, 'turn around' the lives of 120,000 families with multiple problems – such as crime, anti-social behaviour, unemployment and poor school attendance. In 2013, the government announced that the programme would be expanded to support up to 400,000 additional families by 2020. Alongside the EIG (non ring-fenced funding for local authorities to spend on early intervention services needed in their local area), local areas have been able to pool funding for interventions for these families through 'community budgets', as well as access additional funding to trial new approaches. The programme encourages local authorities to: join up local services; deal with problems on a family rather than individual basis; and appoint a single keyworker for families. By March 2015, the programme had reached over 105,000 families. From 2015, the expanded programme will also address families' mental and physical health needs, including substance misuse (Department for Communities and Local Government 2014; and see also guidance for health professionals).[6]

Family and friends care

In 2011, the government issued long-awaited guidance to local authorities on family and friends care (Department for Education 2011). This statutory guidance aims to improve outcomes for children and young people who, because they are unable to live with their parents, are being brought up by members of their extended families, friends or other people who are connected with them. In particular it provides guidance on the implementation of the duties in the Children Act 1989 in respect of such children and young people.

---

6   www.gov.uk/government/publications/troubled-families-supporting-health-needs

Anti-social behaviour

The previous Labour government's programme to tackle anti-social behaviour had a significant focus on parenting. The Crime and Disorder Act 1998 introduced the Anti-Social Behaviour Order (ASBO) and the Parenting Order, since augmented by a number of interventions intended to compel parents to take responsibility for their child's problematic behaviour, whether in a criminal justice, housing or classroom context.

- Acceptable Behaviour Contracts are a 'voluntary' and non-statutory written agreement between a perpetrator of anti-social behaviour and local agencies. As well as outlining behaviour expected of the individual, it can also include a list of what other public agencies should be offering the individual, or in the case of a child, the family, to support a change in behaviour (for example, social services or education welfare).

- Parenting Orders are court orders that require the named parents/carers to attend a parenting programme for up to three months. They can also place requirements on parents to deal with their child's behavioural issues. A breach of this can lead to a fine.

- Parenting Contracts are also 'voluntary' and non-statutory. However, a parent's refusal to agree to one, or failure to abide by its terms, can be cited in court as a reason to make a statutory Parenting Order.

Where these interventions are intended to change the behaviour of the child, good practice would include an assessment of the parent's ability to parent, including identifying parental drug, alcohol or mental health problems. The multi-agency Young Offending Team (YOT) would be able to refer any relevant case to its drug worker or health lead to ensure that a full assessment of the parent's needs could lead to an appropriate intervention.

The coalition government's Anti-social, Behaviour Crime and Policing Act 2014 abolished ASBOs and a number of other measures introduced by the Crime and Disorder Act 1998, replacing them with new measures that aim to restrict the behaviour of those who committed anti-social behaviour while also addressing underlying problems (which could include alcohol or substance misuse or mental health problems). The Act introduced:

- the civil injunction, to stop or prevent individuals engaging in anti-social behaviour quickly, nipping problems in the bud before they escalate. Breach of the conditions of the injunction can result in up to two years in prison for over 18-year-olds and supervision order or civil detention order of up to three months (as a last resort) for 14–17-year-olds

- the criminal behaviour order, which can be served against persons convicted of a criminal offence to prevent the offender from engaging in anti-social behaviour. As with an ASBO, breach of the conditions of the order could result in up to five years in prison for over 18-year-olds and sentencing by the youth courts for under-18s.

Both of these measures can include positive requirements aimed at helping the perpetrator to address the underlying causes of their anti-social behaviour, such as substance misuse.

School absence or truancy

The Education Act 1996 and Anti-Social Behaviour Act 2003 make it clear that parents are obliged to ensure that their school-age children attend school regularly. If they fail to do so, they may be subject to a number of different interventions that can range from an informal interview with the head teacher, through to a more formal interview with an education welfare officer, and on to more punitive measures including Parenting Contracts, Parenting Orders, fines or a community or custodial sentence. Updated guidance on measures relating to parental responsibility for school attendance was published in January 2015 (Department for Education 2015b).

8. Disability

The Equality Act 2010 replaced most existing disability discrimination legislation introduced through the Disability Discrimination Acts of 1995 and 2005. In the 2010 Act, a person has a disability if: they have a physical or mental impairment; and the impairment has a substantial and long-term adverse effect on their ability to perform normal day-to-day activities. Service providers are placed under a duty to make reasonable adjustments to premises or to the way they provide a service to ensure services are accessible to disabled people, and disability is covered under the public sector equality duty, which requires public bodies to eliminate unlawful discrimination and promote equality of opportunity and good relations.

The legal framework for supporting children and young people with special educational needs (SEN) and disabilities is set out in the Children and Families Act 2014 and the *Special Educational Needs and Disability Code of Practice* (Department for Education/Department of Health 2014). Amongst the requirements that this places on local authorities and their partners are:

- providing information and advice for parents and young people
- making joint commissioning arrangements for education, health and care provision for children and young people with SEN and disabilities
- publishing a 'Local Offer', setting out provision they expect to be available across education, health and social care for children and young people in their area who have SEN or are disabled
- drawing up Education, Health and Care Plans for children whose special educational needs are not currently being adequately met by mainstream provision. Local authorities must provide a range of short breaks for disabled

children, young people and their families and set out information about this in the Local Offer.

References

These references are specific to this appendix. Published works cited here and in the main text are listed in the main references section.

Advisory Council on the Misuse of Drugs (2007) *Hidden Harm: Three Years On.* London: Advisory Council on the Misuse of Drugs.

Advisory Council on the Misuse of Drugs (2011) *Hidden Harm: Responding to the Needs of Children of Problem Drug Users.* London: Advisory Council on the Misuse of Drugs.

Department for Communities and Local Government (2014) *Troubled Families Leadership Statement 2014.* London: Department for Communities and Local Government.

Department for Education (2011a) *The Munro Review of Child Protection Final Report: A Child-centred System.* London: The Stationery Office.

Department for Education (2011b) *A Child-centred System: The Government's Response to the Munro Review of Child Protection.* London: Department for Education.

Department for Education (2011c) *Family and Friends Care: Statutory Guidance for Local Authorities.* London: Department for Education.

Department for Education (2015a) *Information Sharing: Advice for Practitioners Providing Safeguarding Services to Children, Young People, Parents and Carers.* London: Department for Education.

Department for Education (2015c) *School Attendance Parental Responsibility Measures: Statutory Guidance for Local Authorities, School Leaders, School Staff, Governing Bodies and the Police.* London: Department for Education.

Department for Education/Department of Health (2011) *Supporting Families on the Foundation Years.* London: Department for Education/Department of Health.

Department for Education/Department of Health (2014) *Special Educational Needs and Disability Code of Practice: 0 to 25 Years.* London: Department for Education/Department of Health.

Department for Work and Pensions (2010) *Universal Credit: Welfare that Works.* London: The Stationery Office.

Department of Health (2013) *Statutory Guidance on Joint Strategic Needs Assessments and Joint Health and Wellbeing Strategies.* London: Department of Health.

Department of Health (2014a) *Care and Support Statutory Guidance.* London: Department of Health.

Department of Health (2014b) *Closing the Gap: Priorities for Essential Change in Mental Health.* London: Department of Health.

Department of Health (2015) *Code of Practice Mental Health Act 1983.* London: The Stationery Office.

Department of Health (England), the Scottish Government, Welsh Assembly Government and Northern Ireland Executive (2007) *Drug Misuse and Dependence: UK Guidelines on Clinical Management.* London: Department of Health (England), the Scottish Government, Welsh Assembly Government and Northern Ireland Executive.

Department of Health and NHS England (2015) *Future in Mind: Promoting, Protecting and Improving our Children and Young People's Mental Health and Wellbeing.* London: Department of Health and NHS England.

Galvani, S. and Forrester, D. (2009) *Social work and substance abuse: teaching the basics.* Southampton: University of Southampton. Available at www.swap.ac.uk/docs/guide-su-learning&teaching.pdf, accessed on 19 October 2015.

Gruer, L. and Ainsworth, T. (2003) *Hidden Harm: Responding to the Needs of Children of Problem Drug Users.* London: Home Office.

HM Government (2008) *Information Sharing: Guidance for Practitioners and Managers.* London: Department for Children, Schools and Families and Communities and Local Government.

HM Government (2010) *Reducing Demand, Restricting Supply, Building Recovery: Supporting People to Live a Drug Free Life.* London: HM Government.

HM Government (2011a) *No Health Without Mental Health: A Cross-government Mental Health Outcomes Strategy for People of All Ages.* London: HM Government.

HM Government (2011b) *Early Intervention: The Next Steps: An Independent Report to Her Majesty's Government Graham Allen MP.* London: HM Government.

HM Government (2012) *The Government's Alcohol Strategy.* London: The Stationery Office.

HM Government (2015a) *Working Together to Safeguard Children: A Guide to Inter-agency Working to Safeguard and Promote the Welfare of Children.* London: The Stationery Office.

HM Government (2015b) *Drug Strategy Annual Review: Delivering Within a New Landscape.* London: HM Government.

HM Treasury (2010) *Spending Review 2010.* London: The Stationery Office.

National Institute for Health and Care Excellence (2011) CG115: *Alcohol-use Disorders: Diagnosis, Assessment and Management of Harmful Drinking and Alcohol Dependence.* London: NICE. Available at: www.nice.org.uk/guidance/cg115, accessed on 16 October 2015.

NHS Commissioning Board (2015) *Safeguarding Vulnerable People in the Reformed NHS: Accountability and Assurance Framework.* London: NHS Commissioning Board.

NTA/Department of Health (2006) *Commissioning and Provision of Treatment for Adult Drug Misusers (MoCAM).* London: Department of Health.

NTA/Department of Health/Home Office (2006) *Models of Care for Treatment of Adult Drug Misusers: Update 2006.* London: National Treatment Agency for Substance Misuse.

Social Care Institute for Excellence (2011) *e-Learning: Parental Substance Misuse.* London: SCIE. Available at: www.scie.org.uk/publications/elearning/parental substancemisuse/index.asp, accessed on 16 October 2015.

Index

23904451R00107

Printed in Great Britain
by Amazon